New Directions in the History of Nursing

This collection of essays demonstrates the international scope of history of nursing scholarship today, encompassing studies from Japan, New Zealand, South Africa, Canada and Europe. The authors examine the social and ethical issues which challenge nurses and midwives in different cultures; the transcultural issues which arise when carers move from one culture to another; and the process of professionalization for women over three centuries. The book highlights the significance of nursing in the history of women's lives and work.

Each chapter contributes to our understanding of the importance of the political world in which nurses and midwives work. Topics covered include: the autobiographies of two Crimean War nurses; the founding of the Norwegian Nursing Association; conflict between nurses/midwives and medical men in eighteenth-century Britain; *sanba* (midwives) and their clients in twentieth-century Japan; professional tensions between doctors and nurses in the USA; industrial action in a mission hospital in South Africa; community nursing in Nazi Germany; the experience of West Indian immigrant nurses in Canada and Britain; the image of nurses through the eyes of British advertisers; and pioneering work by midwives in New Zealand in the twentieth century.

This will make fascinating reading for students and researchers in the history of medicine and nursing, women's history and cultural history.

Barbara Mortimer is a nurse and a historian. She has an extensive network of international contacts among historians of nursing. **Susan McGann** is a historian and has worked in archives for 20 years; she is currently archivist of the Royal College of Nursing of the UK. The editors founded the UK Centre for the History of Nursing in 2000, which has now become the principal focus for historians of nursing in the UK.

Routledge Studies in the Social History of Medicine

Edited by Joseph Melling
University of Exeter and
Anne Borsay
University of Wales at Swansea

The Society for the Social History of Medicine was founded in 1969, and exists to promote research into all aspects of the field, without regard to limitations of either time or place. In addition to this book series, the Society also organizes a regular programme of conferences, and publishes an internationally recognized journal, *Social History of Medicine*. The Society offers a range of benefits, including reduced-price admission to conferences and discounts on SSHM books, to its members. Individuals wishing to learn more about the Society are invited to contact the series editors through the publisher.

The Society took the decision to launch 'Studies in the Social History of Medicine', in association with Routledge, in 1989, in order to provide an outlet for some of the latest research in the field. Since that time, the series has expanded significantly under a number of series editors, and now includes both edited collections and monographs. Individuals wishing to submit proposals are invited to contact the series editors in the first instance.

1. **Nutrition in Britain**
   Science, scientists and politics in the twentieth century
   Edited by David F Smith

2. **Migrants, Minorities and Health**
   Historical and contemporary studies
   Edited by Lara Marks and Michael Worboys

3. **From Idiocy to Mental Deficiency**
   Historical perspectives on people with learning disabilities
   Edited by David Wright and Anne Digby

4. **Midwives, Society and Childbirth**
   Debates and controversies in the modern period
   Edited by Hilary Marland and Anne Marie Rafferty

New Directions in the History of Nursing

International perspectives

Edited by Barbara Mortimer and Susan McGann

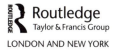

Routledge
Taylor & Francis Group

LONDON AND NEW YORK

First published 2005
by Routledge
2 Park Square, Milton Park, Abingdon, Oxon OX14 4RN

Simultaneously published in the USA and Canada
by Routledge
270 Madison Ave, New York, NY 10016

Routledge is an imprint of the Taylor & Francis Group

© 2005 Barbara Mortimer and Susan McGann for selection and editorial
matter; individual contributors their contribution

Typeset in Times by Prepress Projects Ltd, Perth, Scotland
Printed and bound in Great Britain by TJ International Ltd, Padstow, Cornwall

British Library Cataloguing in Publication Data
A catalogue record for this book is available from the British Library

Library of Congress Cataloging in Publication Data
A catalog record has been requested

ISBN 0–415–30433–4

Contents

Acknowledgements

This book emerged from a conference that took place in the shadow of Arthur's Seat in Edinburgh in July 2000. The conference was planned to celebrate a new millennium and the launch of the UK Centre for the History of Nursing. Our thanks go to all those who attended that conference and particularly to all the contributors to this volume. We are especially grateful to Anne Digby, who first inspired us to consider editing a selection of the conference papers, and to Anne Marie Rafferty, who encouraged us to persevere in our search for a publisher. This volume is the result.

The editors are donating royalties from this book to the UK Centre for the History of Nursing.

Contributors

Anne Digby is Research Professor of History at Oxford Brookes University. She has published widely in the social history of medicine, including *Madness, Morality and Medicine* (1985), *Making a Medical Living* (1994) and *The Evolution of British General Practice* (1999). More recently, she has worked with Helen Sweet on a project examining different forms of medicine in South Africa. Currently she is completing a book on this subject entitled *Medicine, Culture and Society*.

Karen Flynn teaches in the Afro-American Studies and Research Programmes at University of Illinois, Urbana-Champaign. Her research interests include health, migration and the African diaspora. She is also a freelance writer, and writes regularly for *Share*, Canada's largest ethnic newspaper.

Maralyn Foureur is both a midwife and nurse with additional qualifications in psychology, sociology and clinical epidemiology. She received a PhD in epidemiology in 1998 exploring models of midwifery practice and maternity outcomes, and is now actively engaged in clinical midwifery practice, teaching and research. She is the Foundation Clinical Professor of Midwifery and Director of the Collaborating Centre for Midwifery and Nursing Education, Practice and Research at Victoria University, and Capital Coast District Health Board, Wellington, New Zealand.

Mathilde Hackmann graduated as a nurse in 1980 from the Katholische Fachhochschule in Norddeutschland and gained her MSc in nursing and education at the University of Edinburgh. She has worked in a number of hospitals and latterly as a lecturer in nursing and is also an advisor in primary care. She has been a member of the historical nursing research group of the German Association for Nursing Science since 1996 and is currently working as course coordinator and lecturer for continuing education in Hamburg, Germany.

Julia Hallam is a former nurse and health visitor, and now a senior lecturer in the School of Politics and Communications at Liverpool University. She now teaches and researches in the areas of film and television drama. She has contributed to numerous edited collections and journals on aspects of representation, cultural identity and feminist research methodology as well as recent collections on British film and TV drama. Recent books include *Nursing the Image: Media, Culture and Professional Identity* (Routledge 2000) and *Realism and Popular Cinema* (MUP 2000). Currently she is writing a book on Lynda La Plante for Manchester University Press.

Christine E. Hallett is a senior lecturer in nursing at the University of Manchester. She holds the qualifications Registred General Nurse, District Nursing Certificate and Health Visitor's Certificate, and has degrees in Nursing (BNurs, University of Manchester) and History (BA Hons, University of Manchester). She also has PhDs in both nursing education and the history of midwifery. After completing her degree in nursing, she worked for four years as a district nurse and health visitor, before returning to the University of Manchester as a research assistant (1989–1992), principal investigator (1992–1993), lecturer (1993–2004) and senior lecturer.

Aya Homei is currently a Wellcome Research Associate at the Centre for the History of Science, Technology and Medicine, University of Manchester. Her doctoral project involved the re-examination of nineteenth-century Meiji Japan's 'modernization' project by looking at the spheres of medicalized childbirth, childrearing and midwifery. Her publications include '"Normal Birth" and "Modern Hygiene": politics surrounding modern midwife's expertise', *The Japanese Journal of the History of Biology*, 70, February 2003.

Sigrun Hvalvik completed her nurse training in 1982. She was awarded a Master in Nursing Science degree by the Institute of Nursing Science at the University of Oslo in 1996. Her PhD thesis, which she completed in December 2002, was entitled 'Bergljot Larsson and modern nursing' and is a biographical study of the founder of the Norwegian Nursing Association. She is now working as Associate Professor in Nursing Studies, Telemark University College, Norway.

Brigid Lusk is presently an associate professor in the School of Nursing at Northern Illinois University, DeKalb, Illinois. She received her PhD from the University of Illinois at Chicago. Her dissertation, entitled 'Professional strategies and attributes of Chicago hospital nurses during the Great Depression', earned her the 1996 Teresa Christy Award from the American Association for the History of Nursing. She was awarded the 2003 Research Fellowship from the University of Virginia's Center for Nursing Historical Inquiry.

Joan E. Lynaugh is Professor Emerita and Associate Director of the Center for the Study of the History of Nursing, University of Pennsylvania. Her work in establishing the Center has been recognized by the award of many honors over the years. She has published widely on the history of nursing and was the driving force behind the centenary history of the International Council of Nurses *Nurses of all Nations: A History of the International Council of Nurses, 1899–1999*. She has been influential in the nurturing of a new generation of historians of nursing associated with the American Association for the History of Nursing and the Center for the Study of the History of Nursing.

Susan McGann has been the archivist for the Royal College of Nursing since 1986. Her publications include *The Battle of the Nurses* (1992), biographical studies of eight women who influenced the development of professional nursing. She is a co-director of the UK Centre for the History of Nursing.

Barbara Mortimer is a nurse historian and lecturer and co-director to the UK Centre for the History of Nursing. Her PhD in 2002 investigated the careers of private nurses in Edinburgh, Scotland, in the mid-nineteenth century. Her current research interests are in the role of nurses in the history of health promotion.

Julie Fisher Robertson is an associate professor in the School of Nursing at Northern Illinois University. She received her doctorate in educational psychology from Northern Illinois University in 1992. Her research interests include nursing history, nursing practice and policy issues in community settings, student outcomes assessment and critical thinking.

Margaret Shkimba completed an MA in history at York University, Toronto. Her study examined the construction of professionalism in nursing since the Second World War. She is the administrative coordinator of the Women's Health Office in the Faculty of Health Sciences at McMaster University in Hamilton, Canada.

Helen Sweet is a post-doctoral research assistant at the Wellcome Unit for the History of Medicine, University of Oxford. Her current study is the history of medical missions in KwaZulu Natal. She formerly worked with Professor Anne Digby on medical pluralism in the Cape, South Africa. Her particular research interests lie in the social history of nursing and medicine and in oral history. She is founder-convenor of the UK History of Nursing Research Colloquium.

Elaine Thomson holds a degree in history and an MSc in sociology. She received her PhD in the social history of medicine from the University of Edinburgh in 1998. She has published on the development of early physiology and on the practice of medicine by the first and second generations of women doctors in Edinburgh. She is currently a lecturer in marketing at Napier University, Edinburgh, and is working on the history of health promotion in twentieth-century Scotland.

Pamela J. Wood is a registered nurse and historian. She has a BA in social anthropology and history, an MEd and a PhD in history. Her research interests lie in cultural history, particularly the changing meaning of dirt in nineteenth- and twentieth-century public health, nursing and urban development. She is Associate Professor in Nursing in the Graduate School of Nursing and Midwifery at Victoria University of Wellington, New Zealand, and is founder of the History Association of Nursing in New Zealand (HANNZ).

Foreword

Every new volume published in the history of nursing and midwifery presents a moment for reflection and celebration. Since it first attracted critical attention in the early 1980s, the history of nursing has grown steadily into a solid subject of research. I welcome and applaud the current volume as evidence of the strengthening community of scholars, the sustainability of the enterprise and the continued spread of nursing history into new international domains. Significantly, there is continuity with some familiar themes of research: the relationship between nursing and the state, representations of nurses in the media, international influences, the politics of childbirth, conflict with the medical profession, the cultural politics of care. But these are framed within nuanced and textured approaches to analysis demonstrating methodological sophistication in which case studies combine with collaborative, broader survey and epidemiological approaches. Especially heartening is the continued cross-cultural expansion of research into new territory with new contributions from Norway and Japan. Above all, what the present volume reflects is the emerging international support networks and infrastructure for research within nursing and midwifery's scholarly communities. The editors are to be congratulated not only in bringing this volume to fruition but in adding the UK Centre for the History of Nursing to similar endeavours within the Universities of Pennsylvania and Melbourne. Together, these provide important national and international platforms for communication, linkage and exchange between scholars in the field. The next task is to make the history of nursing more competitive and attractive to funders. This will underwrite the future of the field and help it to find a firmer foothold within the academy. Nursing history is no longer a fledgling discipline. Collections such as the present demonstrate it is an energetic and enterprising force to be reckoned with.

Anne Marie Rafferty
London School of Hygiene and Tropical Medicine

1 Introduction

The history of nursing: yesterday, today and tomorrow

Barbara Mortimer

The science, art and craft of nursing, and the nurse 'herself', touch and have touched almost all lives wherever they are lived. Nurses, most of them women, are more numerous than their colleagues who practise medicine. It would seem that the history of nursing is uniquely placed to contribute to the mainstream history of health care and women. Yet nurses and their work have attracted scant attention from historians of medicine and health and, until very recently, from feminist historians. Nurses rarely emerge in accounts of pioneering medicine and were awarded little space in the histories of hospitals.

The written history of 'modern' nursing in the English-speaking world began to be constructed in the second half of the nineteenth century; it rapidly took on the guise of a professional project designed to valorize and justify an emergent profession for respectable women of the time. For many years the creation of a grand narrative of the history of nursing was something engaged with and read almost exclusively by nurses. This position changed only slowly, and in Britain the publication by Brian Abel Smith in 1960 of *A History of the Nursing Profession* marked a new phenomenon, the direction of serious attention to the history of nursing by non-nurses.[1] However, Abel Smith, interested in social policy, made it clear in the introduction to his book that he proposed to write a political history of nursing; he saw himself as unfitted to write 'a history of nursing techniques or of nursing as an activity or skill'.[2] Since 1960, the history of nursing has continued along two tracks. A clear thread of work that valorizes the profession has continued; but a critical historiography emerged in the later twentieth century that is beginning to challenge for a place in the mainstream of social, gender and medical history.

THE BACKGROUND

The history of nursing has been dominated, overshadowed and at times swamped by the iconic figure of Florence Nightingale.[3] Nightingale was an immensely complex, talented and long-lived woman whose published and unpublished output was enormous.[4] Innumerable accounts of her life have been published, and she continues to attract biographers for both a scholarly and a popular readership.

Her official biography, written by Sir Edward Cook with the cooperation of her family, was respectful and included much material from her letters that has been difficult to come by elsewhere.[5] Among many biographies, one by Cecil Woodham Smith has been particularly long lived and continues to be reissued despite serious criticisms from historians.[6] Nightingale's own book, *Notes on Nursing,* has been regularly reprinted[7] and there is an endless market hungry for controversy about this remarkable woman.[8] The singularly powerful image of Nightingale has serious consequences for the historiography of nursing. Her position as, allegedly, first reformer and sole founder of modern nursing has particular impact. Some, overwhelmed by such a powerful figure, find their critical faculties defeated; others, confronted by such authority, fix on single issues and attack the icon with relish. Her unmarried status has invited prurient speculation about her sexuality.[9] It has proved remarkably difficult to award this woman the critical review and assessment that her ability, achievement and reputation deserves.

One device that has supported the legend of Nightingale was the notion of a disreputable nurse of a former era. The figure that embodied this role was fictional, but none the less powerful and influential. Sarah Gamp, created by Charles Dickens and described as addicted to gin and snuff, has been referred to with varying degrees of disbelief, ridicule and amusement by generations since.[10] There have been few attempts to question the veracity of this portrayal.[11] The endurance and widespread acceptance of the image of Gamp as a representative nurse challenges the historian to re-examine the issues thrown up by such a one-dimensional account of a large group of women. Another consequence of the focus on Nightingale has been the virtual exclusion of consideration of nursing prior to the nineteenth century. This imbalance is beginning to be acknowledged and addressed in the work of Carole Rawcliffe and others.[12]

In keeping with a view that turns to Nightingale as a founding icon, the 'modern' history of nursing has derived from Western, Anglo-European culture. As with many other groups in this culture, a favourite device for recording the early history of nurses and nursing has been the creation of institutional histories. These have recorded the great, the good, the admired and the successful from the viewpoint of those individuals. In all circles such histories have been regarded with some suspicion and judged to be both selective and laudatory. Histories of a key institution, the International Council of Nurses (ICN), illustrate the evolution of such accounts in the history of nursing. The earliest history, written by founding members, praised an honourable and proud profession for women; the centenary history, written by historians, strove for balance, and openly discussed the issues raised for the exclusively Anglo-European, and predominantly American, cohort of authors who were writing an international history of nursing.[13] This style of history was very persistent, and as late as 2001 Katrin Schultheiss characterized the history of French nursing as dominated by uncritical institutional histories.[14] However, recent scholars have re-evaluated this collection of relatively uncritical works and now appreciate their value as detailed descriptive accounts that reflect the value systems and the culture of their time.[15]

The valorizing history of nursing attracted small numbers of readers, most of whom were nurses. In response to this small readership there have been a simi-larly small number of broader, contextual accounts of the history of nursing. In the early years two appeared, one by Sarah Tooley, not a nurse, who set out to claim a place for nurses in the imperial project of the most powerful nation of her time.[16] The second was a substantial and scholarly four-volume work by the pio-neering American nurses Adelaide Nutting and Lavinia Dock.[17] Both these texts set out to demonstrate the valuable contribution of women who followed careers in nursing. Both were supported by evidence, Tooley meticulously naming the network of senior women nurses from whom she had gathered her data. Nutting and Dock enjoyed a similarly impressive range of international contacts, but they used the academic device of citing published works to support their arguments and accounts of the history of nursing. These two works show that an anglophone network of women engaged in the construction of this new occupation extended across the Atlantic. The network might appear united. However, the way in which the authors approached the writing of their history hints at differences already deeply embedded in their cultural mindsets and alerts readers to a complex and multilayered history. Following this grand beginning, and continuing until late in the twentieth century, the small number of survey histories of nursing contin-ued to contribute to the construction of a grand narrative.[18] By the late 1980s, a small number of more critical texts appeared in the English-speaking world and more widely.[19] However, in spite of the huge numbers of nurses being trained and educated, there is not a significant demand for new or revised editions of survey histories of nursing. There are clear issues here for historians, social scientists and nurses to consider. How universal is nursing? How important is its history to a profession? How important is the history of such a large female-dominated occupation to historians of gender, health care and medicine?

The opening up of women's history in the 1970s initially had little impact on the writing of the history of nursing.[20] Nurses were certainly a numerically significant group of female workers; however, they seem to have presented an unattractive prospect to researchers, who avoided an occupational group they characterized as inhabiting 'one of the ultimate female ghettos from which women should be encouraged to escape'.[21] In both Britain and North America, this position began to change in the 1980s.

In Britain, the publication of a book of essays in 1980 marked a changing agenda and had a resounding impact. *Re-writing Nursing History,* edited by Celia Davies, a sociologist, represented the first time that a number of mainstream ana-lytic historical and social science approaches were introduced into the study of the history of nursing. In her introduction, Davies made her reasons for publishing the collection explicit; 'our common commitment', she argued, 'is to developing di-verse approaches and questioning an orthodox history of nursing'.[22] In each chap-ter, the authors discussed their chosen theoretical approach. The topics explored in the collection moved into new areas that typified the interests of the new social history. They explored asylum nursing, contrasted nineteenth-century nursing and medical views of nursing 'systems', and investigated traditional women healers. To encourage further research, the collection was completed by a review of archival sources. This book urged nurse historians to seek to locate their work among mainstream accounts in the historical academy, a challenge that was recognized on both sides of the Atlantic.

Other authors applied themes from social history, women's work and the challenges faced by middle-class women to nursing. Martha Vicinus included nursing alongside sisterhoods, higher education, the development of girls' schools and suffrage agitation.[23] The work of Nightingale was addressed using these new tools. Monica Baly made a cool reassessment of the impact of the Nightingale School on nursing and nurse education in Britain and beyond.[24] Anne Summers' account of the origins of female nursing within the British military contributed another thoughtful re-evaluation of Nightingale's position.[25] This work looked beyond Nightingale and recognized a wider context that became clearer when seen through the lens of women's history and social history. Continuity emerged as a theme. The tangle of charitable and religious foundations discernible in the first half of the nineteenth century was interpreted as evidence of early changes in an evolutionary process in which Nightingale played only one part.[26] The work of nurses in the Crimea was scrutinized. Professional 'unreformed' hospital nurses, the new 'lady' nurses and the nursing sisterhoods were all represented in this grim theatre of war. Social class was seen to be of great importance in the early construction of nursing in Britain, an unfashionable theme that has not yet been pursued through to the later twentieth century. The coexistence of diverse approaches to nursing in the late nineteenth- and early twentieth-century hospital began to emerge, approaches that did not depend on a lead from the Nightingale School. Christopher Maggs' study of recruits to general hospital nursing looked beyond the prestigious voluntary hospitals to provincial and unfashionable schools and traced occupational movement among working women who included nursing in their portfolio of skills.[27]

A similar upsurge of scholarship marked the 1980s in the USA. A conference hosted by the Rockefeller Archive Centre in 1981 was influential. Scholars from Britain and the USA, including emerging historians of nursing Barbara Melosh and Susan Reverby, presented papers.[28] The published papers related, in the main, to the USA but included an essay by Davies comparing professionalization in Britain and the USA. Davies drew attention to long-standing and fundamental differences in the mindset of nurses in each country. Her paper also drew attention to cultural differences among nurses within each country; differences linked in both cases to education, economic standing and social class.[29] Also in the USA, the *Bulletin of the History of Medicine* in 1984 marked the changing position in the history of nursing by including a review article by the historian Janet Wilson James. As 'the *Bulletin* has seldom had occasion to examine works in this field', Wilson James provided her readers with a detailed guide and critique of traditional American nursing historiography. She spoke of a profession that 'has had its past to itself', of a 'congealed history', of texts that were 'reflections of the profession's view of itself'. However, she also pointed out a contrasting scenario. She singled out the books of Maggs, Davies and Melosh as work that brought the history of nursing into the historical mainstream and set it in context.[30] The purpose of Wilson James' paper was to introduce the historiography of nursing to a wider readership, in this case to historians of medicine; to make an eloquent plea urging nurses who wrote history to engage with mainstream historical thought. She recognized that the strategy she advocated was already under way.[31]

WOMEN'S HISTORY

The exponential growth in women's history since the 1980s has enriched the context for historical studies of women. As nursing has been a predominantly female occupation, it might appear that the history of nursing would play a significant role in this historical expansion. Many of the dominant themes in women's history have proved to have direct relevance to the history of nursing. The powerful influence of domesticity in the lives of women, including nurses, can be traced in the work of Summers, Vicinus, Melosh, Reverby and others, who recognized that women had to integrate domestic, reproductive and economic roles in their lives.[32] The influence of domesticity extended further. The power of the ordered, middle-class home, supervised and managed by a competent woman, provided a desirable model of social organization: a model that was applied to impose order in disordered situations. Alison Bashford, in her work on the medical professions and sanitary reform, used the domestic model as an explanatory device in her discussion of the struggle for order in public health.[33] The domestic ethos of nursing work and the gender distribution of hospital workers led Eva Gamarnikow to draw an analogy between the patriarchal Victorian family and the gendered structure of the emerging nineteenth-century reformed hospitals. She pointed to the dominant male/father/doctor role, the nurturing female/mother/nurse role and the submissive child/patient role.[34]

One of the key concerns of feminist historians has been to understand the way in which women managed their lives when confronted and surrounded by the social and economic constraints of daily life. The skill with which women negotiated a place for themselves from a position that was often difficult and always sensitive has been attested in accounts of businesswomen, farmers' wives and widows in all walks of life. Yet the contribution that the history of nursing could make to the wider historiography of women is yet to be fully realized. The value of such studies is amply confirmed in Sioban Nelson's account of the lives of religious women, *Say Little, Do Much*.[35] Similarly, debates on separate spheres or the 'public' and 'private' are greatly enriched by Summers' work.[36] Her sensitive reading of Elizabeth Fry's position in the early years of the nineteenth century and her analysis of the difficulties Nightingale and Jane Shaw Stewart endured to occupy public positions nursing the British Army are telling. Each woman had to construct a mode of living that permitted her to engage in such unusual activities and yet to protect her position, status and respectability. Using the work of Habermas, Summers concluded that Fry had the confidence to practise as a Quaker minister because she interpreted her work as belonging to a 'civil' and 'religious' rather than a 'public' sphere.[37] Later in the century, Nightingale and Shaw Stewart, first lady superintendent of female nurses for the British Army

(1861–8), were able to occupy public positions 'under fairly extraordinary conditions . . . neither took a salary, and neither reported to any individual in the official
hierarchy except the Secretary of State for War himself'.[38]

Studies of women's work that draw parallels between women's paid work and
their customary domestic tasks and skills find echoes in the history of nursing. The
analogy can be applied to all household work, including the woman's role as nurse
to the children and sick of her own household. Experience of domestic life differed
among the social classes and women who sought to engage with nursing outside
their own home ranged across the social spectrum. Their varied life experiences
were reflected in different tasks and roles within the nursing world. Traditionally,
hired nurses ranged from rough women engaged as scrubbers in public hospitals
to respectable women who worked as private nurses. When nursing came to be
included as an option for women of higher social status, their special role and skill
as supervisor of a household was transferred to the hospital. Some of these women
were articulate, educated and involved with the suffrage movement, in nursing
they moved into leadership roles.[39] These nurse leaders were the first substantial
group of middle-class women to undertake paid work. Other women who joined
sisterhoods or undertook valuable philanthropic work were unpaid and able to
avoid the taint of working for a salary or wage.[40] Sufficient work has been undertaken to confirm that women who nursed can be located within the wider findings
of the history of women's work. However, the opportunities offered by the study
of such a large group of employed women of varied social standing and in diverse
work places have been underexploited.

Sisterhoods formed a distinctive group of nurses whose work was inspired
by their sense of mission. Throughout the Anglo-European nursing world many
women, lay and religious, spoke of a vocation that they interpreted in Christian
terms. The Anglo-Catholic revival saw the reintroduction of sisterhoods to Britain
and the Irish diaspora saw them transported more widely around the anglophone
world. Since the early controversies of the Anglo-Catholic revival, there have
been many accounts of the sisterhoods. However, as in other areas of historical
scholarship, the nursing sisterhoods customarily attracted least attention. Like the
feminists who avoided nursing 'ghettos', studies of sisterhoods within the church
focused their attention on the teaching and contemplative orders. Insight into this
distinctive group of overtly spiritual women who recognized their own vocation
offers a model to extend understanding of the meaning of vocation and the power
of a spiritual drive among lay nurses and lay women in other walks of life. Recent
revisionist work of sisterhoods in Europe, Australia and North America includes
religious nurses in the wider history of nursing and the even wider context of
health care.[41]

GENDER

The acceptance that nurses are women, and nursing feminine, is one of the embedded assumptions of the history of nursing that should be questioned more
searchingly. There are hints that this is too sweeping an assumption. Margaret

Pelling, speaking of the early modern period, pointed out that there were many masculine work locations – she cited ships, armies, monasteries and mines – where men must have undertaken care.[42] The early Australian colonial experience of a skewed, predominantly masculine, population saw men involved in caring, and Schultheiss noted that in parts of France many men were engaged in nursing.[43] Although some work has been undertaken on the role of men in psychiatric nursing, for example by David Wright and Johnathan Andrews, the position of men in nursing is ambiguous.[44] It is not clear if men have been ejected from nursing or if they undertook a caring role only under the pressure of circumstance; men's studies have yet to make a substantial mark.

In the gendered world of healthcare occupations, the study of nursing or nurses (women) in isolation can begin to seem like a defence mechanism, avoiding the difficulties posed by evaluation of the female contribution in a world dominated by the male. This is an understandable concern for an occupation with its aspirations set on professional status, newly arrived in the 'public' world of work and intent on validating its existence. This criticism could be made of many accounts in the history of nursing. Joan Scott in her essay *Gender: a Useful Category of Historical Analysis* detected three phases in the writing of women's history. First, women were retrieved from obscurity and placed in conventional historical accounts. Second, women were interpreted within the new social history. Both these approaches, in her view, failed to challenge traditional interpretations and established categories of analysis, all of which she saw as imbued with gendered assumptions. Scott welcomed a new third strategy: some researchers who had originally focused their attention on women moved to a wider concern using the notion of 'gender'. By introducing this term, the concept of difference is brought into the analysis. Women, often defined as 'subordinate' or 'oppressed,' are not studied in isolation but their position is sought in relation to others, often their 'oppressors'.[45] It is a measure of increasing maturity in the history of nursing that Bashford's work, which explored the interplay of sanitarian principles, cleanliness, and gender among medical practitioners, deliberately included nurses, medical men, medical women and patients. In the key area of midwifery, formerly a female preserve, predatory masculine *accoucheurs* ultimately overwhelmed midwives. There has been a steady output of work in the history of midwifery yet the diminishing role of female practitioners remains intriguing.[46] In the present volume, Christine Hallett uses a source normally dominated by men – published work – and examines treatises written by women and men that extend our understanding of this crucial area.

The themes that emerged from women's history have proved to be powerful and have emerged at all levels, whether in studies of individuals or of occupational groups. Mary Poovey, a literary scholar, in a study of 'the ideological work of gender' found domesticity infiltrated throughout and chose to describe Nightingale as 'a housewifely woman'. Poovey set out to present a balanced analysis in terms of gender and domesticity.[47] Interpretations that embed the history of nursing in domesticity, and analogies that apply a metaphor of family life, can add value as well as understanding to a fuller history of nursing. However, such interpretations do not suffice for some of the issues that demand attention. The early nurse lead-ers rapidly fixed their eyes on a goal of professionalization, and this issue in the historiography has proved to be spectacularly contentious.

PROFESSIONALIZATION

Arguments about the nuances of meaning and definition of 'profession' have dominated much of the work on the history of occupations. An issue that rapidly emerged was the difficulty of accommodating women in the traditional model. Medicine has been accepted as one of the paradigm professions and its history recognized as an authoritative account of a professionalizing process. It is not surprising that nurses, who worked so closely with medical men, should seek similar recognition for their work. The pursuit of professionalization by nurses has proved to be a long, arduous and at times a rather dispiriting venture. Not sur-prisingly, the search for professional status was an important topic in the earlier triumphalist histories. However, the attempt to position women in a traditional professional scenario proved to be an unrewarding exercise; even attempts to suggest 'semi-professional' status were unconvincing.[48] This dilemma became a tempting area of investigation, and historians and sociologists have weighed in with thoughtful analyses. Of all areas in the history of nursing, this has proved to be one where nursing, a female-dominated occupation, has provided rich material to facilitate crucial investigations of gender issues in social, medical and wom-en's history. The struggle to apply a traditional, male, model of professionaliza-tion to female occupations has been questioned by numerous historians. Linda Hughes doubted this was possible and debated the tensions inherent in an attempt to professionalize domesticity.[49] Davies began to explore the complexity of the concept of profession for nursing in her comparative study of the process among nurses in the USA and Britain.[50] Anne Witz, a sociologist, focused on profes-sional boundaries among medical men and women, nurses and midwives, in a feminist study that distinguished between inter- and intra-professional tensions.[51] Witz responded to the dilemmas and complexities of this professional quagmire by constructing a gender-sensitive model of professionalization. Davies, in her later work, *Gender and the Professional Predicament in Nursing,* presented a particularly telling analysis of the persisting power of gender that first created and then supported assumptions about role and function.[52] She concluded that when embedded in a huge organization, such as the British National Health Service (NHS), these gendered assumptions became all but invisible.

Several of the chapters in the present volume contribute to our understand-ing of the complexity of a history of 'professional' care by women. Brigid Lusk and Julie Fisher Robertson use a journal created by American medical men, the *Journal of the American Medical Association* (*JAMA*), to trace the development of a strengthening and negative view of educated nurses; a group of practitioners who, over time, were increasingly regarded as a threat. In another area of care, Ayah Homei makes a telling analysis of the modernisation and professionaliza-tion of Japanese midwives in the *Meiji* period. Homei admirably unravels the complexities that emerge when additional cultural layers are included with the issues embedded in Western medical professionalization. The modern *shin-sanba* negotiated their professional position in a world influenced by medical men and a government intent on the westernisation of obstetric care. All these developments occurred within a powerful tradition that already included an established birthing culture.

AN INTERNATIONAL AGENDA: RACE AND ETHNICITY

The Anglo-European tradition that was so powerfully represented in the nine-teenth-century history of nursing continues to dominate. This is particularly visible in colonial and post-colonial settings. The 'traditional' Anglo-European model of nursing has remained dominant in the world but the issues raised by the tradition have altered. The ICN, founded by middle-class women in 1899, has remained a significant institution for international nursing. With changing racial profiles among the ICN member states, including the formerly white founding states, a new agenda has become increasingly important. Race and ethnicity are pressing issues for the recent history of nursing. The subject has not yet been addressed in depth within Britain, but in the USA a growing cohort of texts have been written by Afro-Americans and members of other immigrant groups.[53] In South Africa, two studies have tackled the issues thrown up by a post-colonial agenda; one written by a white, the other by a black author.[54] In the present volume, we tackle some of the issues that come out of this increasingly important topic. Helen Sweet and Anne Digby expose some of the racial tensions that were hidden behind the ordered world of a white mission hospital in South Africa in 1949. Their chapter analyses the political and paternalistic power that existed within the field of health care before and during the formal introduction of apartheid in 1948.

Turning to the postcolonial world, issues crowd an agenda that seeks history from the point of view of the colonized.[55] Few have attracted the attention of historians of nursing. In Britain, a long-standing and chronic labour shortage among nurses has resulted in the arrival of successive groups of migrant nurses from Ireland, the West Indies, Mauritius, the former African, and South and South-East Asian colonies. This cultural migration has barely been examined; the countries that accept these migrants have yet to ask the question of why they could not recruit nurses at home to care for their sick countrymen and women; and the complex issues that arise for immigrants, hosts and clientele have hardly been touched. In their chapter in this volume, Margaret Shkimba and Karen Flynn begin to answer these questions from the viewpoint of recent West Indian immigrant nurses in the UK and Canada.

The most dramatic issue confronted by the history of nursing in the past two decades has been scrutiny of the role of nurses under National Socialism in Germany. This subject, long avoided and ignored, was bravely opened up by Hilde Steppe.[56] Since Steppe's early death, the future of the archival materials she had collected has been assured and research in this area continues.[57] Others have followed Steppe's lead.[58] In the present volume, Mathilde Hackmann focuses on one north German region, Osnabrück. She traces the experience of attempts to impose Nazi structures on health care and nursing. A powerful underlying theme in her account is the inevitable paucity of archival sources for research of the topic. Traditional sources have been subject to both the disruptions of war and the vagaries of selective collection or preservation of records for such a sensitive topic. The influence of the National Socialist regime impacted well beyond Germany and resulted in the migration of able men and women who made significant contributions in their new domiciles. Within the UK, this has been noticeably so in nursing.[59] Preliminary work has been done and Professor Paul Weindling has set out to construct the collective biographies of nurses and doctors who came to the UK as refugees, before and during the Second World War, with the intention of assessing the contribution made to the wider nursing and health service.[60]

EDUCATION AND KNOWLEDGE

Nightingale personified the reform of nursing in the nineteenth century, but the action that particularly signified this reform was the founding of a training school. Nurses worldwide lay claim to the Nightingale School as the original model for nurse education. Education as training and the imposition of order symbolized the advance of nursing from a disordered past to a new world peopled by disciplined nurses. Despite an apparently common origin, the educational experience of nurses has differed enormously and owes much to the position of women in different economic, intellectual and gender cultures. Contrasts might be expected between the Anglo-European nations and other parts of the world. However, a significantly different educational climate evolved in Britain and North America. Both professed inspiration from Nightingale. In Britain, schools of nursing were established in hospitals, where nurses were educated in an apprenticeship style. A similar pattern developed widely in the USA. However, for some, education of nurses also represented the sharing and creation of knowledge and American nursing has been represented in higher education since the nineteenth century.[61] In Britain, it was only after the Second World War that nursing was recognized as a discipline that merited inclusion in the universities.[62] In the late twentieth century, without a robust nursing infrastructure in higher education in Britain and elsewhere, those committed to making changes in the intellectual development of nursing education, knowledge and research turned to North American models.[63]

Historians have only recently addressed the nature of the knowledge employed and created by nurses. Anne Marie Rafferty has explored the political history of nursing and the value attached to nursing knowledge in Britain.[64] It is perhaps a simplistic point but, as Rafferty and others have pointed out, in British nursing, changes that might be vigorously advocated by nurses came about only when the wider interests of government and politics coincided with the profession's aspirations. This was famously so regarding state registration, a change introduced in 1919 after over thirty years of lobbying by nurses. The migration of British nurse education to higher education began forty years later and the introduction of student status for learner nurses was not achieved until twenty years after that. The provision of nurse education funding from the NHS budget was finally recognized as anomalous.[65]

More recently, with a strengthening presence of nurses in the universities, the history of nursing research and the growth, evolution and change of nursing knowledge has begun to be addressed. Further work is needed, particularly comparative studies that locate the process of knowledge growth internationally and culturally and distinguish contrasting – perhaps conflicting – and certainly different threads in the growth of nursing knowledge.[66]

NURSING AND THE MILITARY

Nursing and the military has been a strong and confusing theme in the historiography of nursing. Agendas of emancipation, patriotism, heroism and the glorification of sacrifice are all enmeshed in an account that juxtaposes traditional masculine values with a disturbing incursion of the feminine. In Britain since the Crimean war and in the USA since the Civil War (also known as the War Between the States), major conflicts have brought a flurry of activity as women sought a place in the public life of their country, perhaps confusing militarism and patriotism with emancipation. Episodes of war have been followed by the production of artefacts in praise of heroic women. A woman such as Edith Cavell fitted the image of sacrificial heroine so precisely that her memory was commemorated worldwide. A mountain is named for her in Alberta, Canada; a nurse training school in Belgium; and an elegant statue stands outside St Martin in the Fields in London.[67] Yet there has been a selective agenda in the collective memory that records these events. During the Crimean war, Mary Seacole, a black 'doctress', was feted in the British press and a national collection was made for her after hostilities ended. Yet a century later she was barely remembered. During the First World War, women in Britain, the USA and beyond raised huge sums of money to support the work of the Scottish Women's Hospitals in France, Belgium and Serbia. Yet when Leah Leneman and Eileen Crofton wrote about these hospitals at the end of the twentieth century they also had practically disappeared from memory.[68] It seems that what fits the received views survives; it follows that historians of nursing must be alert for alternative histories. Later theatres of war have opened up other themes. In Britain, Penny Starns concluded that militarisation, the inclusion of military procedures and discipline in nursing practices, survived the Second World War and became a feature of postwar British civilian nursing where it posed particular problems. Accounts of Australian and American nurses' contributions to later conflicts continue to tread a difficult path between the glorification of women who dealt with miserable and horrifying experiences, and the need to view such events with the thoughtful detachment of a dispassionate historian's eye.[69]

THE HISTORY OF CARING

In the eyes of many nurses, the most important feature of their science, art or craft has proved to be the most elusive to historians. Many nurses believe that it is the skills of nursing or caring that lie at the heart of their work. The good, skilful or caring nurse is spoken of, yet the nature of the goodness, the skill and the care that is given is hard to define. These are skills honed and exercised in the privacy of the sickroom; they are part of the private experience of illness for the nurse and 'her' patient, and are passed on as part of an oral tradition; something that leaves the merest traces on the written record. Modern-day nurses are still struggling to define and theorize care. Maggs noted the serious limitations of a history of nursing that did not address this issue and attempt to historicize care.[70] He was concerned by a historiography that might be represented as setting out simply to intrude the history of nursing into established historical themes and concluded that 'The world of the nurse, the world of the patient and the world of care remain largely hidden from view.'[71] It is the hidden nature of this history of nursing that makes it so difficult to deal with. Nelson warned that even when this history is glimpsed, interpreting care and caring actions is problematic. Both she and Janet McCalman have commented on an account of nineteenth-century post-operative care in which the skill of the surgeons and the devotion of the nurse resulted in the recovery of a gravely ill patient but damaged the health of the nurse. The nurse cared for her patient day and night and refused to go off duty. They debate the difficulties of interpreting such acts. What do they represent? Was this devoted care that was so punishing to the nurse given by an old style, untrained nurse? Or was she a new style 'trained' nurse? What knowledge did the nurse use? Was this nurse unique? In short, what do these snippets of information tell us of the history of nursing care?[72]

Rafferty traced the beginnings of a history of caring in the writings of Nutting and Dock, who used an ethological model to argue for a biological basis for al-truism and caring.[73] Their suggestion has not been taken up and developed to any great extent, although Marie Françoise Collière, a nurse and historian, has explored the evolution of caring as it moved from care given by women in the home and became systematized as nursing care, given by professional nurses.[74] The dilemmas posed by a concept that is almost invisible and is difficult to evalu-ate in economic terms were considered by Reverby, a historian and not a nurse, in her aptly entitled book *Ordered to Care*. She drew attention to 'a crucial dilemma in contemporary American nursing: the order to care in a society that refuses to value caring'.[75]

Seeking out sources that record care is likely to remain a problem. The direct work of caring was often carried out by the simplest, the lowest, the most menial of attendants, the very people who were unlikely or unable to record their work. The Crimean War marked Nightingale in the popular imagination and saw the creation of personal accounts of nursing. Some of the ladies who took part wrote their memoirs, an action that contributed to the process of building an image of a career fit for ladies and helped to value the activity of nursing or caring.[76] More significant for a history of caring were two accounts that recorded the experience of 'ordinary' yet extraordinary nurses: the (auto)biographies of Elizabeth Davis of Wales and Mary Seacole of Jamaica.[77] The voices of these nurses were re-corded with the assistance of contemporaries who admired them. These accounts resemble oral histories and, in that tradition, they offer a complex, multilayered and richly subjective portrait of the lives, views and experiences of two nurses.

In the present volume, Julia Hallam, in an important piece of work, uses the lens of feminist cultural history to subject these two records to a close analysis. Her model account offers important insights into the meaning of care and caring for these nineteenth-century nurses.

In seeking to create a more recent history of caring, oral history has proved to be a particularly rich source from which the subjective views of practitioners can be captured.[78] In Britain, studies of district nursing by Helen Sweet and Rona Dougall have demonstrated the added value that this research approach offers. The evolution of views, attitudes and understanding can be traced and the meaning to the professionals themselves of elusive concepts such as spirituality and care can be garnered from the practitioners' words.[79] Areas that are usually difficult to access can be made visible through oral history; in particular it is possible to capture multiple views on some topics, interprofessional boundaries being an example.[80]

Another awkward feature that has to be accommodated in the history of caring is the problem posed to the respectable nurse of caring for the sick, damaged, diseased and sexual body of a stranger, activities that involve the management of body fluids and contaminated filth. It was both the gender of the nurse and 'her' involvement with dirt that made pretensions to professional status suspect and unconvincing.[81] One of the first pieces of research to begin to open up this area for enquiry was a sociological study of the nurse's management of the body by Jocalyn Lawler.[82] Lawler concluded that nurses had dealt with dirt deviously, hiding it, disguising it and ignoring it. In a world where the autonomy and power of the professions is repeatedly questioned and subjected to scrutiny, perhaps the analysis and historicisation of the core work of nursing – caring for the disordered body and mind – will attract more attention.[83]

An important response to the complex and sometimes intrusive role of the nurse has arisen because of the activities 'she' carried out. Nursing work required 'her' to invade, physically and emotionally, the private space of others, and has led to the creation of images of the nurse that enabled 'her' patients to deal with the discomfort they experienced as their autonomy was threatened. Seeing the nurse as angel offered comfort and reassurance, the nurse as disciplinarian could become a figure of fun or reassurance, the nurse as erotic sexual object could become a figure of fantasy and mockery. The importance of the image of the nurse over time is attested to in a collection of papers edited by Anne Hudson Jones that traced images of the nurse from the fifth century BCE.[84] More recently, Hallam sought to open out contemporary ideas of the image of the nurse and traced the influence of gender, race and class on professional identity.[85] In the present volume, Elaine Thomson has interpreted the images of nurses as portrayed in advertisements in the nursing press. In this case, we see the nurse on one level as helper and adviser to 'her' client, on a different level as an object to be persuaded by the advertising industry, and on yet another level we might glimpse the nurse's view of herself.

SOURCES

The sources that survive form the foundation of historical study. In the case of nursing, the enormous quantity of material relating to Nightingale sits in stark contrast to the position of other nurses of her time and later. The lives of some nurses were recorded, particularly those who were recognized as 'heroic'. This occasionally makes the construction of a fuller portrait of nurses and nursing possible.[86] However, a consistent theme in the world of the history of nursing is the loss or absence of records. Even distinguished women engaged in formulating and carrying out policy often left no personal papers. It seems that nurses have not perceived their work as having historical importance as a part of the history of women and the history of health care. Susan McGann was repeatedly frustrated by the paucity of papers when preparing her collection of valuable biographical portraits of some key early leaders of British nursing. These portraits open a window into the complexities of women's lives and begin to locate them alongside contemporary medical and administrative men.[87] The scarcity of personal detail for women of this generation stretches beyond the history of British nursing. Many women, significant players in the history of nursing in their own countries and on the world stage, remain largely unknown.[88] In this volume, Sigrun Hvalvik has reconstructed the career of Bergljot Larsson. Larsson was the founder of professional nursing in Norway. Her life, the influences on her thinking and the networks she participated in, could only be reconstructed by a painstaking and international prosopographical exercise that depended as much on collections in Edinburgh as those in Norway.

The scarcity of source material extends beyond the personal papers of individuals. Nursing and nurses were of relatively low status and, despite the immense efforts made by pioneers such as Ethel Bedford Fenwick to found and publish journals, these same journals were not regarded as particularly valuable and very few full runs of the early years of nursing journals survive. In spite of their scarcity, projects to digitize early nursing journals have only recently attracted funding. The single example known at the moment is the *British Journal of Nursing* (1888–1956), published on line by the Royal College of Nursing archives.[89]

The paucity of sources has resulted in the imaginative exploitation of those that survive. Material preserved for different purposes has been exploited to provide an unexpected view of nursing. Imaginative use of sources is reflected in many of the chapters in the current volume. Pamela Wood and Maralyn Foureur have very different interests yet their collaboration has used one source, the records of the St Helens hospital in Wellington, New Zealand, to create two different histories. Wood is in search of a cultural history that uncovers the meaning of the breast and the perineum in the records whereas Foureur, a midwife, traces the empirical and demographic account that is buried in the records.

CONCLUSION

The story told in this chapter is global; it tells of a sophisticated history and historiography of an occupation distinctively marked by its female membership. It is an international history and the work of the nurse is seen as universal. It is also an interdisciplinary history enriched by the contributions of social scientists, feminists and historians of various persuasions. This book embodies these features, rather than offering a comprehensive survey of major themes. It reflects the international nature of nursing and the range of scholarship represented across many countries and cultures. The history of nursing has yet to be written in many settings, and essays that begin to gather together scattered data and answer questions about pioneers are as important as innovative accounts that are pushing out the boundaries in new areas of investigation.

One of the dilemmas of the history of any profession remains for the history of nursing. Who should write this history and who is it written for? Nelson pondered this question at length in her essay 'The fork in the road'. She commented that the traditional readership for the history of nursing, among the alumni of famous hospital training schools, had disappeared. In her view, nursing had found a new catalyst to delineate a professional identity, the creation and expansion of contemporary nursing theory. Maggs also mused about the relationship between nursing theory and the history of nursing. He wondered if the new theories of caring might contribute to a history that did truly examine the history of nursing, i.e. caring, rather than the history of nurses. We do not claim to answer these questions; rather, we would like to focus attention in a slightly different direction. This question has been asked before: Is there something unique about nursing and does a nurse historian bring a particular sensitivity, awareness and insight to the writing of the history of nursing?

Of the seventeen authors in this book, ten have a nursing or midwifery qualification and of those, eight are doubly qualified as nurse (or midwife) and historian. All the chapters make a thoughtful contribution to the history of nursing but it is someone who is doubly qualified who has so creatively addressed the issue of historicising care. The question is not yet closed.

We regard ourselves as privileged to welcome Joan Lynaugh to our group of authors. She has led the way in the changes in the history of nursing in the USA over the past thirty years. She is a nurse and a historian whose achievements go some way to expand on the question we have posed. Along with colleagues, Professor Lynaugh has been a key figure in supporting the AAHN (American Association for the History of Nursing), whose annual conference is supported by international historians and whose journal (*Nursing History Review*) is now established as the major international journal of the history of nursing. Professor Lynaugh has also been instrumental in setting up and raising foundation funds for the Center for the Study of the History of Nursing at the University of Pennsylvania. The Center is attached to the Nursing Department in the University, where Professor Lynaugh followed a career as both an academic nurse and a historian. PhD students in this department are supported in their studies by doubly qualified supervisors who practise as both nurses and historians. In this environment, the questions that are posed and the thinking that goes into them are inevitably informed by both the world of nursing and the world of history.

NOTES

1   B. Abel-Smith, *A History of the Nursing Profession*, London: Heinemann, 1960.
2   Ibid., p. xi.
3   E. V. E. Whittaker, and V. Olesen, 'The faces of Florence Nightingale: functions of the heroine legend in an occupational sub-culture', *Human Organization,* 1984, Vol. 23, pp. 123–30.
4   A project located in the University of Guelph, Canada, is in the process of publishing all Nightingale's known writings. This project has involved searching academic libraries and collections worldwide and has continued, so far, for more than six years: www.sociology.uoguelph.ca/fnightingale/index.htm (accessed January 2004).
5   E. T. Cook, *The Life of Florence Nightingale,* Vol. I *1820–61,* Vol. II *1862–1910,* London: Macmillan, 1913.
6   Reissued most recently in 1996, C. Woodham Smith, *Florence Nightingale,* London: Constable, 1950; see the polite criticism of Greenleaf and the much more astringent comments of Smith: W. H. Greenleaf, 'Biography and the "amateur" historian: Mrs Woodham-Smith's "Florence Nightingale"', *Victorian Studies,* 1959, Vol. III, pp. 190–202; F. B. Smith, *Florence Nightingale: Reputation and Power*, London: Croom Helm, 1982.
7   A useful reprint in 1992 included the full text and a publishing history: V. Skretkowicz (ed.), *Florence Nightingale's Notes on Nursing (Revised, with additions),* London: Scutari Press, 1992.
8   The first seriously critical biography, by Lytton Strachey, appeared in 1918, L. Strachey, *Eminent Victorians,* London: Chatto and Windus, 1918, pp. 117–79.
9   R. Gordon, *The Private Life of Florence Nightingale,* London: Heinemann, 1978 (reissued 2001). More recently, a BBC television programme in 2002 researched by Mark Bostridge resolutely narrowed its focus to present a critical account of Nightingale.
10   C. Dickens, *Martin Chuzzlewit,* London: Chapman & Hall, 1896 (first published in serial form 1843–1844). A leading article in the *Scotsman* newspaper, Edinburgh 16 February 1863, twenty years after she first appeared in print, cited Gamp to summon up an image of the 'old' disreputable nurses.
11   A. Summers, 'The mysterious demise of Sarah Gamp: the domiciliary nurse and her detractors c. 1830–1860', *Victorian Studies,* 1989, Vol. 32, pp. 365–86. B. Mortimer, 'The nurse in Edinburgh c. 1760–1860: the impact of commerce and professionalization', PhD thesis, University of Edinburgh, 2002.
12   Nutting and Dock included study of the earliest times in their comprehensive history and early images of nursing were considered in a collection edited by Anne Hudson Jones. M. A. Nutting, and L. Dock, *A History of Nursing: the Evolution of Nursing Systems From the Earliest Times to the Foundation of the First English and American Training Schools for Nurses,* London: G. P. Putnam and Sons, 1907; N. B. Kampen, 'Before Florence Nightingale: a prehistory of nursing in painting and sculpture', in A. Hudson Jones, *Images of Nurses: Perspectives from History, Art and Literature,* Philadelphia: University of Pennsylvania Press, 1988, pp. 6–39; C. Rawcliffe, *Medicine and Society in Later Medieval England,* Stroud: Sutton Publishing, 1995.
13   M. Breay, and E. G. Fenwick, *History of the International Council of Nurses 1899–1925,* Geneva: International Council of Nurses, 1931; D. C. Bridges, *A history of the International Council of Nurses, 1899–1964: the First Sixty-Five Years,* London: Pitman Medical Publishing, 1967; B. J. Brush, J. Lynaugh, *Nurses of All Nations: A History of the ICN 1899–1999,* Philadelphia: Lippincott, 1999.
14   K. Schultheiss, *Bodies and Souls: Politics and the Professionalization of Nursing in France, 1880–1922,* Cambridge: Harvard University Press, 2001, p. 8.
15   S. Nelson, 'The fork in the road: nursing history versus a history of nursing', *Nursing History Review,* 2002, Vol. 10, pp. 175–88; see p. 180.

16 S. Tooley, *The History of Nursing in the British Empire*, London: S. H. Bousfield, 1906.

17 Nutting and Dock, *History of Nursing*.

18 In Britain, E. S. Haldane, *The British Nurse in Peace and War*, London: J. Murray, 1923; L. R. Seymer, *A General History of Nursing*, London: Faber and Faber, 1932; S. Bingham, *Ministering Angels,* London: Osprey, 1979. For a discussion of the American position see J. Wilson James, 'Writing and re-writing nursing history', *Bulletin of the History of Medicine*, 1984, Vol. 58, pp. 568–81.

19 M. F. Collière, *Promouvoir la vie: de la pratique des femmes soignantes aux soins infirmiers,* Paris: Inter Editions/Masson, 1982; Y. Knibiehler, *Cornettes et blouses blanches: les infirmières dans la société française (1880–1980),* Paris: Hachette litérature, 1984; S. Reverby, *Ordered to Care: the Dilemma of American Nursing 1850–1945,* Cambridge, Cambridge University Press, 1987; R. Dingwall, A. M. Rafferty and C. Webster, *An Introduction to the Social History of Nursing*, London: Routledge, 1988.

20 In Britain, Sheila Rowbotham's book is often used as a marker of the flowering of this new women's history, S. Rowbotham, *Hidden from History: 300 Years of Women's Oppression and the Fight Against It,* London: Pluto Press, 1973. One early work did include nurses in a study of paid work by middle-class women, L. Holcombe, *Victorian Ladies at Work: Middle-class Working Women in England and Wales, 1850–1914,* Newton Abbott: David and Charles, 1973.

21 C. Vance, S. Talbott, A. McBride and D. Mason, 'An uneasy alliance: nursing and the women's movement', *Nursing Outlook*, 1985, Vol. 33, pp. 281–285; see also S. Bunting, and C. Campbell 'Feminism and Nursing: Historical perspectives', *Advances in Nursing Science,* 1990, Vol. 12, pp. 11–24.

22 C. Davies (ed.), *Re-writing Nursing History,* London: Croom Helm, 1980, p. 9.

23 M. Vicinus, *Independent Women: Work and Community for Single Women 1850–1920,* Chicago: University of Chicago Press, 1985, pp. 85–120.

24 M. Baly, *Florence Nightingale and the Nursing Legacy,* London: Croom Helm, 1986; 'The Nightingale Nurses: The myth and the reality', in C. Maggs (ed.), *Nursing History: the State of the Art,* London: Croom Helm, 1987, pp. 33–59. Judith Godden's forthcoming biography of Lucy Osburn, the Nightingale nurse sent to Sydney Hospital to reform nursing in 1868, promises to continue this thoughtful revision, J. Godden, *Lucy Osburn: Purpose and Courage in the Antipodes* (working title, proposed publication 2005).

25 A. Summers, *Angels and Citizens: British Women as Military Nurses 1854–1914,* London: Routledge, 1988.

26 A. Summers, 'The costs and benefits of caring: nursing charities, *c.* 1830–*c.* 1860', in J. Barry and C. Jones (eds), *Medicine and Charity Before the Welfare State*, London: Routledge, 1991, pp. 133–48; 'Elizabeth Fry and mid nineteenth century reform', in R. Creese, W. F. Bynum and J. Bearn (eds), *The Health of Prisoners,* Amsterdam: Rodopi, 1995, pp. 83–101.

27 C. Maggs, *The Origins of General Nursing,* London: Croom Helm, 1983.

28 B. Melosh, 'Doctors, patients, and "Big Nurse": work and gender in the postwar hospital', in E. C. Lagemann (ed.), *Nursing History New Perspectives, New Possibilities,* New York: Teachers College Press, 1983, pp. 157–79; S. Reverby, '"Something besides waiting": The politics of private duty nursing reform in the Depression', in Lagemann, *Nursing History*, pp. 133–56.

29 C. Davies, 'Professionalizing strategies as time and culture bound: American and British nursing *c.* 1893', in Lagemann, *Nursing History*, pp. 47–63.

30 B. Melosh, *The Physician's Hand: Work, Culture and Conflict in American Nursing,* Philadelphia: Temple University Press, 1982.

31 Wilson James, 'Writing and rewriting nursing history'.

32   Reverby, *Ordered to Care*; P. D'Antonio, 'Revisiting and re-thinking the rewriting of nursing history', *Bulletin of the History of Medicine,* 1999, Vol. 73, pp. 268–290.
33   A. Bashford, *Purity and Pollution: Gender Embodiment and Victorian Medicine,* London: Macmillan, 1998.
34   E. Gamarnikow, 'Sexual division of labour: the case of nursing', in A. Kuhn and A. M. Wolpe (eds), *Feminism and Materialism: Women and the Modes of Production,* London: Routledge and Kegan Paul, 1978, pp. 96–123.
35   S. Nelson, *Say Little, Do Much: Nurses, Nuns and Hospitals in the Nineteenth Century,* Philadelphia: University of Pennsylvania Press, 2001.
36   A. Summers, *Female Lives, Moral States: Women, Religion and Public Life in Britain, 1800–1930,* Newbury: Threshold Press, 2000.
37   Ibid., p. 16.
38   Ibid., p. 17.
39   S. Forsyth, 'Nursing leaders and feminist issues: Susan McGahey and the New South Wales experience, 1890–1910', *International History of Nursing Journal,* 1998, Vol. 3, pp. 20–31; S. McGann, *The Battle of the Nurses: a Study of Eight Women who Influenced the Development of Professional Nursing, 1880–1930,* London: Scutari Press, 1992; V. L. Bullough, O. Maranjian Church, A. P. Stein, *American Nursing, a Biographical Dictionary,* London: Garland Publishing, 1988.
40   Frank Prochaska argued that privileged women honed their skills of management and administration by their systematic work as philanthropists. F. Prochaska, *Women and Philanthropy in Nineteenth Century England,* Oxford: Clarendon Press, 1980.
41   S. Mumm, *Stolen Daughters, Virgin Mothers: Anglican Sisterhoods in Victorian Britain,* Leicester: Leicester University Press, 1998; Nelson, *Say Little, Do Much;* S. Malchau, 'Women religious and Protestant welfare. The Sisters of Saint Joseph's Empire of Catholic Hospitals in Denmark', in Y. M. Werner (ed.), *Nuns and Sisters in the Nordic Countries after the Reformation. A Female Counter-Culture in Modern Society,* Uppsala: Studia Missionalia Svecana, LXXXIX (2004).
42   Margaret Pelling, *The Common Lot. Sickness, Medical Occupations and the Urban Poor in Early Modern England,* London: Longman 1998, p. 184.
43   Schultheiss, *Bodies and Souls,* p. 5.
44   D. Wright, 'Asylum nursing and institutional service: a case study of the south of England', *Nursing History Review,* 1999, Vol. 7, pp. 153–70; J. Andrews, A. Briggs, R. Porter, P. Tucker, K. Waddington, *The History of Bethlem,* London: Routledge, 1997.
45   J. W. Scott, 'Gender, a useful category of historical analysis', in J. M. Scott (ed.), *Feminism and History,* Oxford/New York: Oxford University Press, 1996, pp. 152–180, First printed in *American Historical Review,* 1986.
46   There is an enormous literature on the history of midwifery. For this topic see H. Marland and A. M. Rafferty (eds), *Midwives, Society and Childbirth: Debates and Controversies in the Modern Era,* London: Routledge, 1997; A. Wilson, *The Making of Man Midwifery: Childbirth in England, 1660–1770,* Cambridge: Harvard University Press, 1995.
47   M. Poovey, 'A housewifely woman: the social construction of Florence Nightingale', in *Uneven Developments: the Ideological Work of Gender in Mid-Victorian England,* London: Virago, 1989, pp. 164–201.
48   A. Etzioni (ed.), *The Semi-professions and their Organization: Teachers, Nurses, Social Workers,* London: Collier-Macmillan, 1969.
49   L. Hughes, 'Professionalising domesticity: A synthesis of selected nursing historiography', *Advances in Nursing Science,* 1990, Vol. 12, pp. 25–31.
50   C. Davies, 'Professional power and sociological analysis: Lessons from a comparative historical study of Nursing in Britain and the USA', PhD thesis, University of Warwick, 1981.
51   A. Witz, *Professions and Patriarchy,* London: Routledge, 1992.

52   C. Davies, *Gender and the Professional Predicament in Nursing,* Buckingham: Open University Press, 1995.

53   D. C. Hine, *Black Women in White: Racial Conflict and Cooperation in the Nursing Profession 1890–1950,* Bloomington: Indiana University Press, 1989; M. E. Carnegie, *The Path We Tread: Blacks in Nursing Worldwide, 1854–1994,* New York: National League of Nursing Press, 1995; S. L. Smith, *'Sick and Tired of Being Sick and Tired': Black Women's Health Activism in America 1890–1950,* Philadelphia: University of Pennsylvania Press, 1995; C. C. Choy, *'Empire of Care': Nursing and Migration in Filipino American History,* Durham: Duke University Press, 2003.

54   S. Marks, *Divided Sisterhood: Race, Class and Gender in the South African Nursing Profession,* London: Macmillan Press, 1994; T. G. Mashaba, *Rising to the Challenge of Change: a History of Black Nursing in South Afri*ca, Kenwyn: Juta & Co., 1995. See also: A. Digby, and H. Sweet, 'Nurses as culture brokers in twentieth-century South Africa', in W. Ernst (ed.), *Plural Medicine, Tradition and Modernity, 1800–2000,* London: Routledge, 2001, pp. 113–29.

55   For South Asia see, for example, J. Gourlay, *Florence Nightingale and The Health of the Raj,* Aldershot: Ashgate, 2003.

56   Only Steppe's articles have been published in English; as yet her books have not been published in translation. H. Steppe, 'Nursing under totalitarian regimes: the case of National Socialism', in A. M. Rafferty, R. Elkan and J. Robinson (eds), *Nursing History and the Politics of Welfare,* London: Routledge, 1997, pp. 10–27; H. Steppe, *Krankenpflege im Nationalsozialismus,* Frankfurt: Mabuse-Verlag, 2001.

57   These are now lodged in the Hilda Steppe Archive in the Library of the Fachhochschule, Frankfurt am Main: www.fh-frankfurt.de/wwwbibl/07/dokpfle.htm (accessed January 2004).

58   See, for example, C. Schweikardt, ' "You gained honor for your profession as a brown nurse": the career of a National Socialist nurse mirrored in her letters home', *Nursing History Review,* 2004, Vol. 12, pp. 121–38.

59   J. W. Stewart, 'Angels or aliens? Refugee nurses in Britain, 1938 to 1942', *Medical History,* 2003, Vol. 47, pp. 149–72.

60   Interviews have been carried out with doctors. As yet the planned interviews with nurses have not been undertaken.

61   The first professor of nursing in the USA was appointed in1895 at the University of Texas and qualified nurses were admitted to Teachers College, New York, in 1899. By 1923 the Goldmark Report was able to state confidently that 'many' universities in the USA had graduate courses in nursing.

62   The first academic department of nursing in a British university was in Edinburgh in 1956. Rockefeller funding was an important factor in enabling this initiative. R. Weir, *A Leap in the Dark: the Origins and Development of the Department of Nursing Studies, the University of Edinburgh,* Penzance: Jamieson Library, 1996. The transfer of all nurse education to the tertiary sector was completed only by 2000.

63   A. M. Rafferty, 'Nursing: an intellectual culture', paper presented at the 40th Anniversary Celebrations of the Department of Nursing and conferment of an Honorary Fellowship of the University of Edinburgh upon Winifred Logan Gordon, 1996.

64   A. M. Rafferty, *The Politics of Nursing Knowledge.* London: Routledge, 1996.

65   British nurse education was funded by the Department of Health and the 'student' nurse was treated as an employee. This situation resulted in increasingly awkward problems and anomalies.

66   P. D'Antonio, 'Toward a history of nursing research', *Nursing Research,* 1997, Vol. 46, pp. 105–110.

67   A. E. Clark-Kennedy, *Edith Cavell: Pioneer and Patriot,* London: Faber and Faber, 1965. Cavell was brought up in Swardeston near Norwich. The website maintained by the rector gathers many images of Cavell together: www.edithcavell.org.uk (accessed January 2004).

68   L. Leneman, *In the Service of Life: the Story of Elsie Inglis and the Scottish Women's Hospitals*, Edinburgh: Mercat Press, 1994; E. Crofton, *The Women of Royaumont, a Scottish Women's Hospital on the Western Front*, East Linton: Tuckwell Press, 1997.

69   C. Enloe, *Does Khaki Become You?*, London: Pluto Press, 1983; J. Bassett, *Guns and Brooches: Australian Army Nursing from the Boer War to the Gulf War*, Melbourne: Oxford University Press, 1997; P. Starns, 1997 'Military influence on the British civilian nursing profession 1939–1969', 1997, PhD thesis, University of Bristol; P. Starns, *Nurses at War: Women on the Front Line 1939–45*, Stroud: Sutton Publishing, 2000; Minerva, *Quarterly Report on Women and the Military*; this journal reports an upsurge in activity relating to the role of female nurses and the military.

70   C. Maggs, 'A history of nursing: a history of caring', *Journal of Advanced Nursing*, 1996, Vol. 23, pp. 630–5.

71   Ibid., p. 633.

72   S. Nelson, 'A history of small things', in J. Latimer (ed.), *Advanced Qualitative Research*, Oxford: Blackwell Publishing, 2003, pp. 211–30; J. McCalman, *Sex and Suffering, Women's Health and a Women's Hospital: the Royal Women's Hospital Melbourne 1856–1996*, Melbourne: Melbourne University Press, pp. 76–8.

73   A. M. Rafferty, 'Writing, researching and reflexivity in nursing history', *Nurse Researcher*, Vol. 5, pp. 5–16.

74   Collière, *Promouvoir la vie*; M. F. Collière, Invisible care and invisible women as health care providers', *International Journal of Nursing Studies*, 1986, Vol. 23, pp. 95–112.

75   Reverby, *Ordered to Care*, p. 1.

76   Sr. M. Aloysius, *Memoirs of the Crimea*, London: Burns and Oates Ltd, 1897; M. Nicol, *Ismeer or Smyrna and its British Hospital in 1855*, London: James Madden, 1856; F. M. Taylor, *Eastern Hospitals and English Nurses*, two vols, London: Hurst and Blackett, 1856.

77   Z. Alexander and A. Dewjee (eds), *The Wonderful Adventures of Mrs Seacole in Many Lands*, Bristol: Falling Wall Press, 1984 (first published 1857); J. Williams (ed.), *The Autobiography of Elizabeth Davis: Betsy Cadwaladyr: a Balaclava Nurse*, Cardiff: Honno, 1987 (first published 1857).

78   J. Bornat, R. Perks, P. Thompson and J. Walmsly (eds), *Oral History, Health and Welfare*, London: Routledge, 2000.

79   R. Dougall, 'Perceptions of change: an oral history of district nursing in Scotland 1940–1999', PhD thesis, Glasgow Caledonian University, 2002; H. Sweet, 'District nursing in England and Wales *c*.1919–1979, in the context of the development of a Community Health Team', PhD Thesis, Oxford Brookes University, 2003.

80   There are many examples in widely different settings, see for example, J. E. Lynaugh and J. Fairman, *Critical Care Nursing: A History*, Philadelphia: University of Pennsylvania Press; Schweikardt, ' "You gained honor for your profession as a brown nurse": the career of a National Socialist nurse mirrored in her letters home', *Nursing History Review*, 2004, Vol. 12, pp. 121–38.

81   Bashford examined dirt and public health; Pamela Wood focused on colonial dirt. Bashford, *Purity and Pollution*; P. Wood, 'Constructing colonial dirt: a cultural history of dirt in the nineteenth century colonial settlement of Dunedin, New Zealand', PhD thesis, University of Otago, Dunedin, New Zealand, 1997.

82   J. Lawler, *Behind the Screens: Nursing, Somology and the Problem of the Body*, Edinburgh: Churchill Livingstone, 1991.

83   Professional authority has been thoroughly questioned in the later twentieth century, and the waxing and waning of professional power has been explored by Harold Perkin, concluding with his book *The Third Revolution*. H. Perkin, *The Third Revolution: Professional Elites in the Modern World*, London: Routledge, 1996.

84   A. H. Jones (ed.), *Images of Nurses: Perspectives from History, Art, and Literature*, Philadelphia: University of Pennsylvania Press, 1988.

85   J. Hallam, *Nursing the Image: Media Culture and Professional Identity,* London: Routledge, 2000.

86   Sister Dora – Dorothy Pattison – was the subject of a sentimental biography by her former student Margaret Londsale, *Sister Dora: A Biography*, London: C. Kegan Paul & Co, 1880. A later biographer commented on the value of this text. It was the only source of accounts by Sister Dora's patients of the nurse's care. J. Manton, *Sister Dora: the Life of Dorothy Pattison*, London: Methuen, 1971. Agnes Jones, a graduate of the Nightingale Training School, sent to 'reform' nursing in Liverpool died, in post, of fever. Her heroic work was recounted in E. L. Courtenay, *Agnes Jones*, London: Religious Tract Society, 1871.

87   McGann, *The Battle of the Nurses.*

88   A welcome essay examined one aspect of the career of an influential figure in German nursing, Agnes Karll. A thorough examination of the careers of Karll and other German nurses is awaited. G. Boschma, 'Agnes Karll and the creation of an independent German Nursing Association, 1900–1927', *Nursing History Review,* 1996, Vol. 4, pp. 151–68.

89   This journal was founded and for many years edited by Fenwick herself: www.rcn. org.uk/historicalnursingjournals (accessed January 2004). This project was funded by the Wellcome Trust's Research Resources in Medical History Grants Scheme.

2 Ethical lives in the early nineteenth century

Nursing and a history of caring

Julia Hallam

Autobiographies and biographies of nurses can be found on the shelves of many public libraries in Britain. Written for a general readership, many of these accounts contain detailed descriptions of the day-to-day practicalities of living and working as a nurse in various spheres of professional practice. What might these (auto)biographies contribute to our knowledge of nursing history? Christopher Maggs argues that nursing history helps furnish the detail of political, economic and social history but has yet to generate its own conceptual statements about nursing and caring.[1] It is almost as though history and nursing are separate, and that studies of the history of nursing bear no relationship to theories about nursing or caring. Maggs is interested in how an exploration of the historical landscape might aid the construction (reconstruction and destruction) of nursing or caring models. He suggests that if nursing history is to contribute to the development of nursing knowledge, we have to investigate 'the world of the patient and the world of care [that] remain[s] largely hidden from view'.[2] This study explores the contribution nursing (auto)biographies can make to what Maggs productively suggests might be termed a history of caring by revealing not only the institutional and social development of nursing as a profession but the skills, knowledge and ethos of everyday nursing practice.

(Auto)biographies are a potential source of what Patricia Benner terms 'expert testimony'.[3] By collecting accounts of nursing practice from 'expert nurses' – those who spend their working lives engaged in the practical aspects of nursing – Benner suggests it is possible to begin to establish what nurses do when they nurse and examine the ways in which they practise caring. (Auto)biographical accounts can contribute to this project by constructing a history of nursing vested in the experiences of those who worked as nurses. Many popular (auto)biographies were written in the twentieth century, and some in the Victorian era, when the Nightingale reforms began to be instituted (albeit unevenly) throughout the British Isles and further afield as nursing began its struggle to become recognized internationally as a profession. A minority of these accounts bear substantial reference to the pre-Nightingale era, of which two, *The Wonderful Adventures of Mrs Seacole in Many Lands* and *The Autobiography of Elizabeth Davis: Betsy Cadwaladyr, a Balaclava Nurse*, are perhaps the most well known in Britain. These accounts form the focus of this enquiry.[4]

This chapter is divided into five sections; the first focuses on theoretical and methodological approaches to the study of (auto)biography developed by feminist researchers interested in (auto)biography as a way of mapping a submerged history of female experience. The second briefly outlines definitions of the ethics of care as it is used within nursing to identify and illuminate ways in which concepts of caring are used in these (auto)biographical texts. Section three focuses on the contextual discourses that shaped these (auto)biographies, mapping the relationship between white middle-class formations of female respectability and the effect these have had on constructions of the caring self as it is represented in the two accounts. Section four focuses on articulations of nursing skill and knowledge expressed in the texts and their relationship to an ethics of care. Finally, the usefulness of the exercise is assessed: can a deconstructive critical approach to (auto)biographical texts offer any fresh insights into early and mid-nineteenth-century concepts of nursing and caring?

WORKING WITH (AUTO)BIOGRAPHIES

(Auto)biographies are a rich source of information about women's lived experience but, like all written accounts and records, they need to be treated with some caution as sources of the truth of that experience. Feminist researchers, with their avowed intention to excavate and map the contours of women's lives, have pointed out some of the theoretical and methodological problems of working with (auto)biographies. Particular attention is given in their analyses to the forms of expression in which the self is represented. (Auto)biographies often demonstrate a degree of feminist political awareness of the self as a speaking subject and appear to offer unmediated access to the truth of individual experience; however, this truth can be questioned on both theoretical and material grounds. From a theoretical point of view, (auto)biography is a form of writing tied to fictional conventions such as narrative (hence the common use of travel and travel metaphors to structure life stories) and the notion of closure, or completion. The life story is often articulated as a linear tale of development, growth and maturation, and is inevitably tidied up in the interests of making a coherent impression on the reader. Feminist social historian Elizabeth Wilson has summed up the dilemma of how to evaluate (auto)biography quite succinctly: ' . . . all autobiography is in some sense fictional – the remembrance or the searching again for the "lost times" is never just an act of memory or research, but is inevitably a re-creation, something new'.[5]

Writers of (auto)biographies can strive to present truthful accounts of lives and selves, but their project is inevitably compromised by the very nature of writing as a creative, imaginative activity and the structuring of experience into forms of narrative and narration that can be easily understood.

At a more practical level, writers have some control over the ways and means (both aesthetic and institutional) through which representations of the self are constructed and materialize. Unlike more personal accounts, such as journals and diaries usually written for self consumption (perhaps with the idea of recording events for posterity), published (auto)biographies are written with a particular reading public in mind. The (auto)biographies analysed here were written in the immediate aftermath of the Crimean War and sought, in different ways, to cash in on the wave of public sentiment and support for those at the front that followed in its wake. Mary Seacole, a Jamaican doctress and nurse, is well known today as one of the first black women to be recognised for her contribution to nursing history.[6] Elizabeth Davis (Betsy Cadwaladyr), a working-class Welsh woman, is perhaps less well known than she deserves to be given that low-status women in Britain at that time found it very difficult, because of their class, to leave any public record of their lives. Seacole wrote her autobiography to appeal to the philanthropic sensibilities of a middle- and upper-class readership; she hoped to convince readers of her worthiness so that they would send her enough money to resolve her bankruptcy problems. The recorder of Elizabeth Davis' oral testimony – the Welsh historian Jane Williams – realized the topicality and significance of her story when she met Davis after her return from the Crimea in 1856. A researcher of patterns of Welsh economic migration, Williams' interest in recording Davis' life story was stimulated by the nurse's severe criticisms of Nightingale's control of resources. Williams recorded and edited a series of interviews with Davis, which were first published in 1857, again with the ostensible purpose of raising funds to care for Davis, whose health and strength were destroyed by her work in the Crimea.

Seacole and Davis were accustomed to the vagaries of fortune, having spent their younger lives living as independent, single women travelling the world. Seacole, the daughter of a free black Jamaican doctress and hotelier, was a successful business woman as well as a nurse and healer well known and admired for her work among high-ranking British military officers. Accounts of the time refer to her as a doctress, nurse and a sutler; her medical skills were learnt from her mother, who ran a boarding house in Jamaica patronized mainly by military families.[7] The family was well-off by Jamaican standards, belonging to a class of mixed-race people termed in the legal language of the day 'mulattos'. Like all free black people, they had few civil rights; they could not vote or hold public office; inheritance was limited and there were also restrictions on land ownership. However, many were well educated, some women engaged in trade, others hired themselves as domestic servants or worked in one of the many hotels owned by black women. At the outbreak of war in 1853, Seacole sailed from Jamaica to England to offer her services to the Nightingale cause; unable to secure an appointment as a nurse, she undertook to finance her own trip to the front. Entering into business with a distant relative, she set up the equivalent of an officer's mess for the wealthier soldiers in the Crimea. When the war ended abruptly in March 1856, Seacole was left with expensive redundant stock and no market for the goods and equipment she had laid in. She returned to London impoverished and facing bankruptcy charges. Her autobiography, first published in 1858, has to be read bearing in mind its ostensible purpose: to raise money to off-set the debts incurred as a result of borrowing money to fund her work on the battlefields.

Davis was part of a large migrant workforce of Welsh women who left their homes to enter domestic service in England. The daughter of a non-conformist clergyman, her early years were spent on a hill farm; when she was five years old her mother died. Davis was sent to live in the household of their landlord where she learnt domestic skills, reading, writing and English. Aged fourteen, she left Wales for Liverpool and became a servant, the only occupation available at that time to a respectable girl of her class. After many years spent in domestic service, a role that often blurred the boundaries between housekeeping, cooking, cleaning, nursing and caring, she read of the battles in the Crimea in newspapers and, determined to offer her services to the cause, she joined a party of nurses under Miss Stanley.

These two accounts are particularly interesting in terms of articulating an ethics of care because, unlike most other women who served as nurses in the Crimea, neither belonged to a religious order nor came from a privileged background.[8] They were popular accounts about significant contemporary events written to appeal to a Victorian upper-middle-class readership and, as such, they sought to place in the foreground those values that would warrant the writer to be considered 'deserving' of financial support by their affluent readers. These books tell us as much about the economic value of respectable femininity and its relationship to caring as they do about the moral constitution of mid-nineteenth-century society and its attitudes to women. Their accounts of nursing and caring probe the vocational model of an ethics of care rooted in notions of duty and self-sacrifice found in official histories of nursing such as those by Brian Abel-Smith and Monica Baly.[9] For Seacole and Davis, responsibility for the health and well-being of others is an integral aspect of their gendered socialisation in small, comparatively isolated communities. The treatment of disease and ill-health is a skilful practice based on inherited knowledge and experience as well as a caring activity with an ethical dimension.

THE ETHICS OF CARE

Caring has long been claimed as a concept at the heart of nursing, sometimes described as the thing that distinguishes nursing from other professions. Care is increasingly recognized as the moral foundation, ideal and imperative of nursing.[10] What counts as caring at any particular historical moment is highly dependent on context; meanings of care are historically contingent and change over time. Caring is not just a subjective and material experience but one in which particular historical circumstances, ideologies and power relations create the conditions under which caring can occur, the forms it takes and the consequences it will have for those who undertake it.[11] Ethical selves are shaped by social discourses that situate care in relation to broader formations of gender, religion, class and ethnicity as well as factors such as age, nationality and physical location.

Given that caring as an activity is shaped by a range of historically contingent factors, any attempt to define it is fraught with difficulty. For the purposes of analysis, I have drawn on definitions of the ethics of care developed from the work of Nel Noddings, Benner and Judith Wrubel.[12] Caring is a response to stress, it is a form of coping, of helping those in distress or suffering from dis-ease; nurses care by relieving stress, distress and dis-ease. Increasingly, nurses are establishing ethical principles and guidelines for practice that differentiate the ways in which nurses care from everyday caring activities. The ethics of care is appealing to nurses and nursing theorists partly because it seems to offer a different way of doing things from mainstream (bio)ethics, partly because it is linked to feminism (and nursing continues to be a female-dominated profession) and partly because of the belief that care is in some way central to nursing.[13] Peter Allmark points out that it is not simply that nurses care – everyone does – rather it is the objects of their care and the way it is expressed that are of importance. Per Nortveldt suggests that when nurses care for patients, moral value is intrinsic to both observation and professional performance; as a nurse looks, so she or he discovers various pathophysiological phenomena that are not purely factual and of neutral value.[14] A nurse's observation is invested with value because the observation has a bearing on evaluating the patient's distress, which ascribes moral importance to his or her human condition; what affects the patient most affects the nurse too as an obligation. Nursing knowledge (epistemology) and its essence in being-with-the-other (its ontology) is fundamentally related to being-for-the-other, to being responsible for the other, being answerable to their pain and vulnerability (its ethics).

How might nurses' (auto)biographies express these finer distinctions?; how might these writers articulate a sense of 'being-for-the-other'? It is important to examine the text not only for descriptive accounts of the ways in which these writers claim they treat and care for others, but to determine how they articulate their own response to distress and suffering in combination with acknowledging responsibility for the well-being of the other. Arguably, this aspect of caring has a gendered dimension. In the early 1980s, Carol Gilligan controversially claimed that females and males have different responses to moral issues.[15] In tests with young people, she found that females solved ethical problems differently to males, with females taking account of the emotional impact of decisions on family and friends. Males took a more pragmatic, materialist approach and sought clear outcomes to ethical dilemmas in terms of financial compensation or legal retribution. She concluded that women develop an 'ethics of care', the underlying logic of which is a psychological logic of relationships that contrasts with the generally male formal logic of fairness that informs the justice approach. Although this research has been challenged on the basis of its essentialist assumptions, it remains generally accepted that there are gendered differences in the moral make-up of males and females.[16] Some explanations for this hinge on psychological theories but, as Gilligan herself suggests, there are also social causes. Joan Tronto argues that women's different moral expression might be a function of their subordinate or tentative social position.[17] Research with members of minority cultures in the USA, such as African-Americans, Chicano and Inuit peoples, indicates a greater concern with moral issues and a foregrounding of virtues associated with the ethics of care such as commitment, generosity, compassion and respect for others. If, as Tronto suggests, the caring self is not only a product of socialized gender difference but, as other nursing theorists such as Margaret Dunlop suggest, associated with subordinate social status, this has some implications for the ways in which we think about caring historically, and how a history of caring interacts with the history of nursing.[18]

THE CONTEXT OF CARING

The ethics of care articulated by Seacole and Davis in their (auto)biographies is an integral aspect of mid-nineteenth-century discourses of Western femininity, discourses predicated on middle-class ideals of female respectability that are intricately embedded into social relations between women and between men and women, as well as between people of different classes, creeds and ethnicities. Although it is now generally acknowledged that religious values played a vital role in re-constructing nursing as a respectable profession for women, and that many lower middle-class women who became nurses later in the century did so in pursuit of a respectable life,[19] the influence of discourses of respectability on earlier constructions of nursing and nurses has received less sustained attention. Indeed, the portrait of the drunken Sairey Gamp in *Martin Chuzzlewit* by English novelist Charles Dickens is often regarded as emblematic of the pre-Nightingale nurse. Neither Seacole nor Davis belonged to a religious order but both considered themselves religious and, according to their own accounts, led ethical lives that culminated in caring for the sick and injured on the battlefields of the Crimea. In spite of numerous opportunities to marry both women chose to live their lives as single, independent women at a time when to do so was considered scandalous. Seacole states categorically that 'it was from a confidence in my own powers, and not at all from necessity, that I remained an unprotected female'.[20] Seacole and Davis preferred to defy social convention and remain in control of their own lives, a decision regarded by many in society as tantamount to living a disreputable life.

Marriage and family were central to definitions of female respectability in the early nineteenth century. The rising middle classes ascribed special qualities of a moral and ethical nature to women, which defined the domestic sphere as their principal area of responsibility and operation. This is sometimes referred to as 'woman's mission': women were expected to use their special qualities as a reforming influence on family and friends, and to donate their leisure time and energy to societies engaged in social and moral reform. One of the contradictions of 'woman's mission' is that it regulated the distance between women of different social classes. Linda Nead discusses the way the phrase was used to describe the role of the respectable woman in the reclamation of 'the fallen' (prostitutes and other women of dubious morality), and the way that the term differentiated between the 'deserving' and 'undeserving' poor.[21] Within this context, 'respectability' was not only an indication of social status but also of moral value and social worth.[22]

Philanthropic work also constructed hierarchical relationships between white women and those of different races. Vron Ware argues that it was a short step from bestowing charity on poor (deserving) women to applying the same principles of compassion to assist and plead for those who were enslaved, a more abstract group of poor with whom white middle-class women had little physical contact. Abolishing slavery was a political struggle aimed at changing hearts, minds and laws. The abolitionist movement allowed women to use their image of respectability in the public sphere but the success of the campaign was followed, paradoxically, by an increase in British imperial control of many areas of the world. The relationship between white women and those of different races evolved throughout the nineteenth century; middle-class women participated in British colonization as missionary workers, nurses and teachers, and they married colonial officials. This expanded the reach of 'woman's mission' way beyond their own 'urban jungles' to many parts of the world.[23]

Nineteenth-century racialist thought intertwined science, religion and aesthetics, 'defining Aryans or Caucasians as the pinnacle of the human race in every respect', including physical beauty.[24] Non-white peoples were associated with dirt, with bodily emissions and body odours considered distasteful to the 'civilized' sensibilities of white middle-class Victorians.[25] Anne McClintock argues that self-definition of the middle classes, with their emphasis on taste, respectability and the cult of domesticity, was central to maintaining the imperialist project: categorizations of race were interlocked with those of class through the generic definition of 'dangerous classes'.[26] Working-class women are distanced from 'taste', from the static, silent, invisible and composed forms of conduct and behaviour that were deemed hallmarks of respectability.[27] White middle-class femininity was defined as the ideal but also as the most passive and dependent of femininities. In contrast to the frail physical bodies and 'delicate' temperaments of middle-class women, working-class women were paradoxically coded; on the one hand, they were depicted as inherently healthy, hardy and robust, on the other they were seen as a source of infection and disease, in part the result of their 'dangerous' sexual appetites.

Elizabeth Davis' familiarity with these discourses is apparent throughout the text; for example, she refers to the unsuitability of middle- and upper-class women for nursing work because of their frail dispositions, emphasizing her own physical prowess and strength, accompanied by an honest nature and dependable character:

> I do not undervalue the services of any of the ladies, but real, highborn gentle-women are not accustomed to hard manual labour, and are not strong enough for it. In performing servile offices they put constraint upon themselves, and hurt the feelings of the men, who are acutely sensible of the unfitness of such work for persons of high station. Ladies may be fit to govern but for general service, persons of a different class, who could put their hands to anything, were more useful.[28]

In her introduction to a recent edition of Davis' autobiography, historian Deirdre Beddoes describes Davis as a physically striking woman possessed of a remarkably strong personality, characterized by enterprise, courage, honesty, a great sense of adventure and an enormous capacity for hard work.[29] Davis was brought up in a Welsh society where social class created fewer barriers between people than in urban England, but nonetheless she is acutely aware of the discourse of respectability and constructs a distance between herself and 'unruly' or disreputable women based on interpretation of character and readings of appearance. She says this of the other nurses chosen with her to go to the Crimea:

> I am sure the committee of ladies in England did all they could to procure good nurses for the Eastern hospitals; but they were obliged to take other people's recommendations, and could not know enough of the working classes to judge for themselves. Many women, therefore, were sent out as nurses who had never filled any position of trust before, and were really incapable of the duties they had undertaken . . . Some among them, too, were persons of unsteady habits, who, not doing well at home, hoped to fare better abroad.[30]

Davis is aware that, in spite of their well-intentioned efforts, the philanthropists had very little knowledge of or contact with working-class women; the rigid social hierarchy prevented any communication between women of different classes.

Mary Seacole, coming from quite a different place and background, grew up with a similar awareness of differences among women. In 1850, at the age of forty-five, having developed a reputation for her doctoring skills, she left Jamaica to join her brother in New Granada, a journey she made alone, protected only by her servants. One consequence of her actions was that she lost any remaining vestiges of respectability in the eyes of her contemporaries. Describing her situation in South America, she comments:

> My present life was not agreeable for a woman with the least delicacy or refinement . . . the females who crossed my path were as about as unpleasant specimens of the fair sex as one could well wish to avoid . . . only this, if any of them came to me sick and suffering (I only say this out of simple justice to myself). I forgot everything, except that she was my sister, and that it was my duty to help her.[31]

Judged by the standards of the day, the women she extends her care to were 'undeserving' prostitutes; she justifies her care of them by drawing on concepts of family, an image that draws on the protestant ethics of care that evokes the familiar notion of 'woman's mission' to her readers. She uses this discourse to position herself as a 'deserving' woman, someone who has acted charitably to 'undeserving' others and therefore worthy of receiving charitable assistance herself.

Seacole was aware of racial prejudice and disliked white Americans for the racist attitudes they displayed in South America. The Crimean War began in 1853; Seacole sailed to England to offer her services to the Nightingale cause only to find her offer of service rejected. She becomes aware that the racist attitudes she discovered among white Americans were shared by the English; she was not only the wrong class, but also the wrong colour:

I was so conscious of the unselfishness of the motives which induced me
to leave England – so certain of the service I could render among the sick
soldiery, and yet I found it difficult to convince others of these facts . . . Did
these ladies shrink from accepting my aid because my blood flowed beneath
a somewhat duskier skin than theirs? Tears streamed down my foolish cheeks
. . . tears of grief that any should doubt my motives.[32]

She tries to excuse their racial prejudice saying 'in my country where people
know our use it would have been different'.[33] Unable to secure an appointment as
a nurse, she undertook to finance her own trip to the Crimea and offset the costs
of providing medical and nursing care by setting up the equivalent of an officer's
mess for the wealthier soldiers. Unlike many sutlers, she ran a clean house where
gambling and drunkenness were strictly forbidden. She was known for relieving
suffering among the troops, taking mules laden with medicine, drinks and food to
the heart of the battle lines, as well as running daily surgeries for all and sundry
from her collection of huts known as the British Hotel.

Seacole and Davis were adventurers who spent their lives travelling the world;
both were accustomed to dealing with all manner of diseases, tropical illnesses
and injuries. Above all, both were working women who managed their own financial affairs at a time when few women managed to live their lives independently
of men. Both depended in part on trading medicinal and nursing skills as a means
of earning a living, both took pleasure in developing their knowledge of sickness
and disease and both considered caring an integral aspect of their practice. Their
autobiographies afford some insight into how gender interacts with differences
of class, race, nationality and religion to create 'ethical subjectivities': the ethical
self. How that ethical self is constructed textually and represents a concept of
nursing practice focused on caring through the processes of 'being-for-the-other'
is the focus of analysis in the following section.

NURSING KNOWLEDGE, SKILLS AND CARING

Analysing the ethics of care in this context depends upon considerations of empathy *and* judgement, emotion *and* rationality as a whole person response to the
realities of 'the other's' suffering, pain and discomfort. The texts were analysed
initially for their descriptions of nursing skills and knowledge; then particular
phrases that pertain to personal beliefs, attitudes and values in relation to these
activities were isolated. What is particularly notable in the following extracts is
the degree of personal responsibility exercised by Davis and Seacole in making
decisions about the treatment of those they care for; feeling responsible for how
others are feeling, both physically and mentally, is integral to their concept of
care. This is not merely a matter of empathy, of understanding distress and feeling sympathy or acting compassionately; Seacole and Davis use their skills and
understanding of sickness to actively intervene on behalf of the other.

Seacole describes herself as driven by a yearning for medical knowledge and a
burning desire to help her fellow beings:

I do not deny (it is the only thing indeed that I have to be proud of) that I am pleased and gratified when I look back upon my past life, and see times now and then, places here and there, when and where I have been enabled to benefit my fellow-creatures suffering from ills my skill could often remedy.

I am not ashamed to confess – for the gratification is, after all, a selfish one – that I love to be of service to those who need a woman's help . . . I ask no higher or greater privilege than to minister to it . . .[34]

The satisfaction Seacole gains from her work is presented as personal rather than altruistic; she is not driven by feelings of religious duty or service, only by her own satisfaction and the fulfilment she gains from helping those in need of care. She claims to have inherited a desire to learn and practice medical skills from her mother:

My mother was, like many of the Creole women, an admirable doctress . . . It was very natural that I should inherit her tastes; and so I had from early youth a yearning for medical knowledge that has never deserted me.[35]

In addition to learning her mother's skills she studied with naval and military surgeons who stayed under her roof, becoming skilled in the surgical treatment of wounds.

Shortly after arriving in South America, an outbreak of cholera tested Seacole's skills to their limits:

There was no doctor in Cruces . . . I was obliged to do my best . . . I went hastily to the patient and at once adopted the remedies I considered fit. It was a very obstinate case, but by dint of mustard emetics, warm fomentations, mustard plasters on the stomach and the back, and calomel, at first in large then in gradually smaller doses, I succeeded in saving my first cholera patient in Cruces.[36]

She understood the necessity for the sick room to be clean and well ventilated, isolated her patients to prevent the spread of disease and gave them relief by administering 'warm fomentations' and 'mustard plasters', treatments based on the same principles as those in use in hospitals before the introduction of antibiotics. In addition, she used her surgical skills to tend knife and gunshot wounds.

Seacole's yearning for medical knowledge drives her to investigate the effects of disease on the body and the efficacy of her treatments by performing autopsies on those who die of infectious diseases:

I began to think . . . that if it were possible to take this little child and examine it, I should learn more of the terrible disease which was sparing neither young nor old, and should know better how to battle with it.[37]

As she becomes older and more experienced, her faith and confidence in her own skills and abilities grows:

> So strong was the old impulse within me that I waited for no permission . . . lightly my practised fingers ran over the familiar work, and well was I rewarded when the poor fellow's groans subsided into a restless uneasy mutter . . . I stooped down and offered some tea to his baked lips . . .[38]

Unafraid of authority, possessed of courage, determination and considerable initiative, she pursues her quest to use her knowledge and skills, always accompanying palliative action with sensitivity to her patients' response. She is acutely aware of how medical treatments affect people differently: 'One great conclusion . . . that the course of treatment that saved one man would, if persisted in, have very likely killed his brother'.[39] She treats people holistically, caring for each person as a unique individual.

Elizabeth Davis articulates a similar use of initiative and resourcefulness in coping with and caring for sick people, drawing on a combination of knowledge, skills and experience. Employed as a servant to a sea captain and his family, she describes how she manages an unexpected confinement at sea:

> I found her very ill and having tried hot flannels, hot salts and other things in vain, I began to recollect that I had formerly seen a person in that state before. I also thought over what I had read in Dr Buchan's book, and became quite certain about the case. I gave her a cup of green tea, which had wonderful effects, and about two in the morning, a fine boy was born – I being the sole attendant on her and the infant.[40]

During the course of her various employments, Davis taught herself to read shipboard medical manuals, combining this knowledge with her own observations. She uses this experience on further voyages: 'Fourteen women were confined during the voyage and I assisted the surgeon in attending them'.[41]

Davis offers several accounts of where her role as servant collapses into that of a nurse; she cares for her sick employers in much the same way that she might care for a member of her own family. Their faith in her abilities is articulated in the following extracts:

> I did all I could for him and watched him day and night. High fever came on, he became delirious and raving. He would suffer no one but me to come near him. I could not keep him in his bed . . . I got together all the doctors of the town to attend him; but they did him no good. I feel sure that the one who was first with him did not understand his disorder, and mistreated it.[42]

Davis articulates a sense of confidence in her knowledge and abilities through her assessment of the situation, caring for the man until he dies:

When I had nursed him for a week, he became sensible again, lay very quiet, and told me of his affairs . . . Two hours afterward I looked at him. He was lying very still, and I saw that he was altered, his face was ghastly, and his features sharpened. As I bent over him, he breathed one short sigh and was gone.[43]

She is also accustomed to dealing with accidents:

. . . my master was brought home to London, propped up with pillows in a coach. He was impatient to come, thinking he should get well the sooner for my nursing. His back had been injured by the fall and his health was affected also by the shock. He was very ill; but with great care, he revived and quite recovered in the course of time.[44]

Although her accounts often lack detailed descriptions of her actions, a sense of being-for-the-other is conveyed in the importance she attaches to acting on careful observation: 'I know that the lives of many poor fellows were saved by careful attention in feeding and nursing them night and day. Many must have died without proper attendance at night.'[45] Davis is aware that only vigilant, knowledgeable nursing care can save their lives.

Both women know that the prevention of disease is equally important as its treatment and possess a wide knowledge of all forms of food and drink and their relationship to a healthy diet:

I went there to fish and occasionally to gather oranges, lemons, pomegranates, grapes and other fruit. I ate so many of these that people used to say the fruit was the means of saving me from fevers and other diseases of the country. I used to bring back with me my boat full of fruit for the ship's crew and passengers.[46]

In the Crimea, Davis' ability to prepare nourishing food and drinks for large numbers of people from the meagre resources available was quickly recognized by her superiors, 'Mother Eldress established me in the kitchen, and gave me entire charge of it. She said she saw I could do well, and could trust me.'[47] Seacole personally prepared all the food and drinks served at the British Hotel as well as making her own remedies from the stock of herbs and medicines she had brought with her from England.

During the course of their working lives, Seacole and Davis often risked their own health and sometimes their lives to try and prevent the suffering and death of others. Seacole recounts how she finds herself in a remote area, the only source of medical and nursing care during an outbreak of plague:

. . . for a few minutes I felt an almost uncontrollable impulse to run out into the stormy night, and flee from this plague spot . . . and then, with the aid of the frightened women, I applied myself to my poor patients. I stayed with them until midnight, and then got away for a little time . . . I was tired to death. I found the worst cases sinking fast.[48]

On the battlefields of the Crimea, she was renowned for taking medicines and refreshments into the heat of the battle to attend the injured:

> I left my horse in charge of some men, and with no little difficulty, and at no little risk, crept down to where some wounded men lay, with whom I left refreshments.[49]
>
> I hastened to the scene of the action, anxious to see once more the faces of those who had been so kind to me in life. That battlefield was a fearful sight for a woman to witness.[50]
>
> I attended to the wounds of many French and Sardinians and helped to lift them into the ambulances. . . I derived no little gratification from being able to dress the wounds of several Russians.[51]
>
> I dressed the wound of one of its officers, seriously hit in the mouth; I attended to another wounded in the throat, and bandaged the hand of a third, terribly crushed by a rifle bullet.[52]

Seacole ministers to the sick on the battlefield irrespective of social and national differences, political allegiances and dangers to herself. Davis similarly places her own health and well-being at risk during her time at the Crimea, caring for people according to their needs:

> It was no time to save oneself when so many were suffering. The patients, officers and all used to call me 'Mother', always behaved to me with respect, and said they were grateful to me. Many have told me since that they owed their lives to the care I took of them.[53]
>
> My health became very bad. The atmosphere of the hospital was unhealthy and everybody saw that I had been working too hard. I suffered from diarrhoea and dysentery.[54]

Her health and strength broken by the long hours and poor working conditions, Davis died three years after her return to England.

CONCLUSION

The ethics of care articulated by these (auto)biographies has a strong Christian ethos, as might be expected from accounts designed to appeal to the charitable inclinations of an upper-middle-class mid-nineteenth-century readership, but neither of the ethical selves constructed in these texts is motivated to care solely by religious duty or altruism. Religion seems less a spiritual focus than a means of national and social self-identification; neither woman discusses her religious affiliation or practice in any depth or detail. Susan Reverby points out that in the past caring has been associated with duty, with subservience and with altruism.

Nursing was organized under the expectation that its practitioners would accept a duty to care rather than demand a right to determine how they would satisfy this duty: 'Because nurses have been given the duty to care, they are caught in a secondary dilemma: forced to act as if altruism (assumed to be the basis for caring) and autonomy (assumed to be the basis for rights) are separate ways of being.'[55] Seacole and Davis avoid this dilemma: although altruism does play a role – both in its later, secular sense of doing one's duty out of concern for others and in its earlier, religious sense of sacrificing the self for a higher ideal – they nurse partly from economic necessity, but not least because of the opportunities it offers to exercise judgement and independence of thought. Most importantly, both determine *how* they satisfy their desire to care, which is seen only in part as a duty. Of the time she worked as a nurse at a London hospital, Davis says this:

> Having been much accustomed to the sick, and to all sorts of casualties, I engaged myself, as a nurse, at Guy's Hospital, and continued there for some time – perhaps a year. The doctors, finding me steady and sober, wanted me to become a night nurse, in place of one who behaved ill. This I refused, and thereupon left the hospital. I next took to nursing private patients, being recommended by surgeons and physicians to whom I was well known . . . I did not like nursing so well as being in service . . .[56]

Davis finds domestic service preferable to nursing because of the relative autonomy in her work and increased opportunities to exercise skills and knowledge based on her own judgement rather than the dictates of others.

Davis and Seacole combine knowledge, skills and being-for-the-other in their practice, seeking to alleviate distress and disease and deriving personal satisfaction and fulfilment from their work. They are 'expert' nurses, highly skilled practitioners whose ethics of care depend on a similar range of characteristics that we might identify today. Benner argues that much of the decision making conducted by expert nurses is derived from an intuitive response based on experience, where the on-going effect of responding in a good way builds the repertoire of ethical response. In this model, rational deliberation is only necessary in the case of ethical breakdown or in the case of conflicting and competing values. Principles, of themselves, are unable to produce expert ethical behaviour, which evolves only from practice, 'in familiar but problematic situations, rather than standing back and applying abstract principles, the expert deliberates about the appropriateness of his [sic] intuitions.[57] Davis and Seacole articulate a similar attitude to care guided by their ethical response to each person as a unique individual, a response that combines knowledge and experience, rational assessment and intuitive action.

The ethics of care are part of the virtue ethics, the appeal to qualities of character, like courage, generosity, commitment and responsibility. Verena Tschudin outlines caring as a relationship in which compassion, competence, confidence, conscience and commitment are mobilized by the care-giver to promote the health and well-being of those in need of care.[58] MacIntyre emphasizes the cultivation of virtues such as courage, wisdom, prudence, temperance, caring, honesty and responsibility.[59] Davis and Seacole articulate their life stories through a moral framework that situates themselves as 'virtuous'. Their accounts privilege personal characteristics such as bravery, respect for others, loyalty, honesty, compassion, wisdom and selflessness. Neither pursues knowledge for its own sake or primarily for financial gain, although both depend on their work to earn their living. Seacole runs a system whereby those who can afford to pay do so, subsidizing the treatment of those who cannot:

> It must be understood that many of those who could afford to pay for my services did so handsomely, but the great majority of my patients had nothing better to give their doctress than thanks.[60]
>
> I cannot conscientiously charge myself with doing less for the men who had only thanks to give me, than for the officers whose gratitude gave me the necessities of life.[61]

She treats and cares for all comers, irrespective of class, creed or ethnicity or their ability to pay, '. . . willingly had they accepted me, I would have worked for the wounded in return for bread and water',[62] as does Davis '. . . making no difference, but giving care and attention to whoever was in the greatest need, whether officers or men'.[63] The texts can be read as a plea that virtue should be rewarded in this world as well as in the next.

Davis died three years after the publication of her autobiography, her own health and strength broken by her experiences at the Crimea; her financial situation is unknown. Seacole's health was also damaged but she was much feted on return; *The Times*, for example, questioned the attentions lavished on Nightingale, testifying to Seacole's 'courage, devotion, goodness of heart, public services and great losses undeservedly incurred'.[64] In 1856 *Punch* published a poem in her honour; the following year the officers she had helped held a military benefit to raise funds to meet her debts. Popular admiration ensured her book was a best seller.[65] She prospered in her old age, died twenty-five years later and was largely forgotten until the centenary of the Crimean War, when the Jamaican Nurses Association elected to name their new headquarters after her.

Of particular interest to nursing history are the ways in which Seacole and Davis actively integrate nursing and medical knowledge, practical skills and caring into being-for-the-other in a society where working women were expected to serve others, to obey commands and to follow orders. The ethical lives led by these two women present exemplary models of caring; they make care more visible as something to be valued both as a virtue and as a principle. They also add to our concepts of caring the vital elements of personal rights and pleasures; one hundred and fifty years later, these accounts continue to resonate with heartfelt passion for their work. The pleasure and personal fulfilment found in actively exercising knowledge, skills and being-for-the-other tend to be omitted from most contemporary models of the ethics of care; it is this legacy that Davis and Seacole contribute to our understandings of care as the moral foundation, ideal and imperative of nursing.

NOTES

1   C. Maggs, 'A history of nursing: a history of caring?' *Journal of Advanced Nursing,* 1996, Vol. 23, pp. 630–5.
2   Ibid., p. 631.
3   P. Benner, *From Novice to Expert: Excellence and Power in Clinical Nursing Practice,* Menlo Park, CA: Addison Wesley, 1984.
4   Z. Alexander and A. Dewjee (eds), *The Wonderful Adventures of Mrs Seacole in Many Lands,* Bristol: Falling Wall Press, 1984; J. Williams (ed.), *The Autobiography of Elizabeth Davis: Betsy Cadwaladyr, a Balaclava Nurse,* Cardiff: Honno Press, 1987.
5   E. Wilson, 'Tell it like it is: women and confessional writing', in S. Radstone (ed.), *Sweet Dreams: Sexuality, Gender and Popular Fiction,* London: Lawrence and Wishart, 1988, p. 21.
6   The word black is used here as a political descriptor to refer to peoples of the African diasporas.
7   Alexander and Dewjee argue that this local knowledge of herbal medicine and midwifery was based on that brought from Africa and used by black women on the plantations. Alexander and Dewjee, *Wonderful Adventures,* p. 13.
8   Most other (auto)biographical accounts of nursing and related activities during the Crimean War were written by upper-class women or those with strong religious affiliations: see, for example, Sister Mary Aloysius, *Memories of the Crimea,* London: Burns and Oates, 1897; Lady Alicia Blackwood, *A Narrative of Personal Experiences and Impressions During a Residence on the Bosphorus Throughout the Crimean War,* London: Hatchard, 1881; Margaret Goodman, *Experiences of an English Sister of Mercy,* London: Smith Elder and Company, 1862; Mrs Tom Kelly, *From the Fleet in the Fifties,* London: Hurst and Blackett, 1902. Robert Richardson has edited the journal of Sarah Terrot, R. Richardson (ed.), *Nurse Sarah Anne: with Florence Nightingale at Scutari,* London: John Murray, 1977. There are also numerous historical accounts of the activities of different religious groups such as the Sisters of Mercy.
9   B. Abel-Smith, *A History of the Nursing Profession,* London: Heinemann, 1975; M. Baly, *Nursing and Social Change,* London: Heinemann Medical, 1980.
10   M-J. Johnstone, *Bioethics: a Nursing Perspective,* 2nd edn, Marrickville: Harcourt-Brace, 1994, p. 132.
11   S. Reverby, 'A caring dilemma: womanhood and nursing in historical perspective', *Nursing Research,* 1987, Vol. 36, p. 5.
12   N. Noddings, *Caring: a Feminine Approach to Ethics and Moral Education,* Berkeley: University of California Press, 1984; P. Benner and J. Wrubel, *The Primacy of Caring: Stress and Coping in Health and Illness,* Menlo Park, CA: Addison Wesley, 1989.
13   P. Allmark, 'Is caring a virtue?' *Journal of Advanced Nursing,* 1998, Vol. 28, p. 466.
14   P. Norveldt, 'Sensitive judgement: an inquiry into the foundations of nursing ethics', *Nursing Ethics,* 1998, Vol. 5, pp. 385–92.
15   C. Gilligan, *In a Different Voice,* Cambridge, MA: Harvard University Press, 1982.
16   For a critique within a nursing context, see, for example, A. Lipp, 'An enquiry into a combined approach for nursing ethics', *Nursing Ethics,* 1998, Vol. 5, pp. 122–38.
17   J. Tronto, 'Beyond gender difference to a theory of care', in M. J. Larrabee (ed.), *An Ethic of Care: Feminist and Interdisciplinary Perspectives,* New York/London: Routledge, 1993, pp. 240–57.
18   M. Dunlop, 'Is a science of caring possible?' in P. Benner (ed.), *Interpretive Phenomenology: Embodiment, Caring, and Ethics in Health And illness,* San Francisco: Sage, 1994, pp. 27–42.
19   See, for example, M. Vicinus, *Independent Women: Work and Community for Single Women 1850–1920,* London: Virago, 1985; and A. Simnett, 'The pursuit of respectability: women and the nursing profession 1860–1900', in R. White (ed.), *Political Issues in Nursing: Past, Present and Future,* Vol. 2, Chichester: John Wiley and Sons Ltd, 1986, pp. 1–23.

20 Alexander and Dewjee, *Wonderful Adventures*, p. 61.
21 L. Nead, *Myths of Sexuality: Representations of Women in Victorian Britain*, Oxford: Blackwell, 1988, pp. 196–7.
22 B. Skeggs, *Formations of Class and Gender: Becoming Respectable*, Thousand Oaks, CA: Sage, 1997, pp. 100–101.
23 V. Ware, *Beyond the Pale: White Women, Racism and History*, London: Verso, 1992, p. 109.
24 R. Dyer, *White,* London: Routledge, 1997, p. 71.
25 Dyer points out that associations between spirituality and cleanliness are prominent in the writings of protestant reformer Martin Luther. Ibid., p. 75.
26 A. McClintock, *Imperial Leather: Race, Gender and Sexuality in the Colonial Context,* London: Routledge, 1995.
27 L. Davidoff, 'Class and gender in Victorian England', in J. L. Newton, M. P. Ryan and J. R. Walkowitz (eds), *Sex and Class in Women's History*, London: Routledge, 1983, pp. 17–71; E. Stanley, *The Diaries of Hannah Cullwick*, London: Virago, 1984.
28 Williams, *Elizabeth Davis*, p. 173.
29 Ibid.
30 Ibid., p. 162.
31 Alexander and Dewjee, *Wonderful Adventures*, p. 100.
32 Ibid., p. 126.
33 Ibid., p. 124.
34 Ibid., p. 78.
35 Ibid., p. 56.
36 Ibid., p. 77.
37 Ibid., p. 81.
38 Ibid., p. 142.
39 Ibid., p. 83.
40 Williams, *Elizabeth Davis*, p. 54.
41 Ibid., p. 61.
42 Ibid., p. 150.
43 Ibid.
44 Ibid., p. 147.
45 Ibid., p. 183.
46 Ibid., p. 125.
47 Ibid., p. 172.
48 Alexander and Dewjee, *Wonderful Adventures*, p. 80.
49 Ibid., p. 196.
50 Ibid., p. 197.
51 Ibid., p. 203.
52 Ibid., p. 208.
53 Williams, *Elizabeth Davis*, p. 181.
54 Ibid., p. 196.
55 Reverby, 'A caring dilemma . . .', 1987.
56 Williams, *Elizabeth Davis,* p. 152.
57 Unpublished manuscript by Dreyfus, Dreyfus and Benner quoted in L. Wros, 'The ethical context of nursing care of dying patients in critical care', in P. Benner (ed.), *Interpretive Phenomenology: Embodiment, Caring, and Ethics in Health and Illness*, San Francisco: Sage, 1994, pp. 255–77, quotation p. 269.
58 V. Tschudin, *Ethics in Nursing: the Caring Relationship*, Oxford: Butterworth Heinemann, 1992.
59 A. MacIntyre, *After Virtue,* Notre Dame, IN: University of Notre Dame Press, 1984.
60 Alexander and Dewjee, *Wonderful Adventures*, p. 79.
61 Ibid., p. 173.
62 Ibid., p. 135.

63 Williams, *Elizabeth Davis*, p. 178.
64 'While the benevolent deeds of Florence Nightingale are being handed down to posterity with blessings and imperishable reknown, are the . . . actions of Mrs Seacole to be entirely forgotten, and will none now testify to the worth of those services of the late mistress of Spring Hill?' (*The Times*, 24 November 1856).
65 Alexander and Dewjee, *Wonderful Adventures*, pp. 30–1.

3 Bergljot Larsson (1883–1968), founder and leader of the Norwegian Nursing Association

A case study of the influence of international nursing

Sigrun Hvalvik

On 24 September 1912, Bergljot Larsson called in 'sisters' from the whole of Norway to discuss the establishment of an association for educated nurses. A few hours after the meeting took place, the Norwegian Nursing Association (NNA) was born, one of the last nursing associations to be founded in Scandinavia; Finland, Denmark and Sweden had already established their organizations. The decision to found the NNA was not made overnight. The idea was conceived not long after Larsson started to work as a nurse and was nurtured during her stay in Scotland from 1909 to 1911. By the time she attended her first international nursing congress, at Cologne in August 1912, preparations in Norway were almost complete. In the processes that led up to the final establishment of the NNA, inspiration, ideas, knowledge and support were provided by a range of individuals and institutions both within and beyond Norway. Larsson was the first president of the NNA, a position she held for twenty-three years.

This chapter argues that Larsson's formative work experience abroad, and her professional contact with European nursing leaders, informed the initiative she took in founding the NNA. Her experiences abroad were also of great significance for her further actions as a leader of the organization. In the first part of the chapter, priority is given to the period of her life passed in Edinburgh. During her stay in the Scottish capital, she met members of the British women's movement and supporters of the British campaign for state registration. These encounters contributed to the creation of her fundamental views regarding women and nursing. The ways in which these views or visions were nurtured during her stay are also traced. In the last part of the chapter, a further argument is proposed that Larsson's visions were crucial for the founding of the NNA itself, and influenced the issues and projects she promoted during her time as leader. As regards her contact with European nursing leaders, it is proposed that these contacts provided practical insights and the encouragement she needed to transform her visions and ideas into the reality of the NNA.

THE STARTING POINT

When Larsson left Norway in 1909 'to study nursing in Edinburgh', an expression she used herself, she was twenty-six years old. After a one-year training course in

1905–6, she worked as a nurse in the medical wards of the municipal hospital of Kristiania (Oslo).[1] In 1907 she established the first nursing union in Norway for the nurses working at the same hospital.[2] By the time she left for Edinburgh, the demand for nurses in Norway reflected the variable conditions of nursing education then available. Only a small number of nursing schools offered a training course of more than one year and among those to benefit from training courses after 1868 were the deaconesses, the first trained nurses in Norway. Deaconesses, skilled and unskilled nurses worked side by side in all areas. They all experienced low wages, hard work and long working days. However, increasing attention was paid to trained nursing at this time and Norwegian doctors took an active part in establishing nursing education. They also expressed admiration for, and were inspired by, progress in British and Danish nursing.[3] Nurses themselves looked abroad and, from the end of the nineteenth century, several nurses travelled to England, Scotland and Germany to study nursing.

Larsson stayed in Edinburgh for two years and three months. Her first experiences were gained at the City of Edinburgh Fever Hospital, where she took a one-year 'fever course'. For fifteen months from January 1910 she practised as a nurse on different wards in the Royal Infirmary of Edinburgh (RIE).[4] During her stay in Edinburgh, activities related to both the women's movement and to the campaign for state registration were much reported in the press in Great Britain.

THE WOMEN'S MOVEMENT

When Larsson arrived in Edinburgh in 1909, women's suffrage was very visible. The Edinburgh Women's Suffrage Society was established the year she arrived and the suffragettes held well-publicized meetings and processions, making the status of women an issue that could not be ignored. The militant suffragettes received publicity through activities that led to arrests and, among those imprisoned, hunger strikes in custody.[5] In Scotland generally there was considerable activity among women and a very active suffrage milieu existed in Edinburgh, in which the female doctors were particularly involved.[6] Larsson later maintained that the suffragettes impressed her while she was in Edinburgh. Their vision assigned women new positions and was grounded in a belief that women's particular qualities were of crucial importance for the creation of a better society. Women's inherent qualities, then most often described and recognized in the domestic sphere, should receive wider recognition. The debates around the role of women had considerable influence on the development of Larsson's views of women and her thoughts about their potential future role in society.

Larsson's interest in the women's movement and in the ideas it promoted was further strengthened through two special women who became her role models when she was in Edinburgh. These were Ethel Bedford Fenwick, an international figure, and Annie Gill, Lady Superintendent at the Royal Infirmary of Edinburgh. At the time, Mrs Fenwick was the leader of the national campaign for state registration for nurses. In addition, as the founder and President of the International Council of Nurses (ICN), an organization that had its origin in the International

Council of Women (ICW), and her involvement in the women's movement, Fenwick forged strong links between this movement and nursing.[7] Miss Gill was one of Mrs Fenwick's supporters in the campaign for registration. By embracing Mrs Fenwick's position, Miss Gill also embraced the radical and intellectual wing of nursing in Great Britain, the group whose connections with international nursing and the suffragette movement were strongest. Larsson's close contact with Miss Gill when she worked at the Royal Infirmary of Edinburgh strengthened her belief in women and in their importance for the further development of 'the good society'.

Women's issues also received great attention in the *British Journal of Nursing* (*BJN*), the official organ for several important nursing associations. The journal was owned and edited by Mrs Fenwick and it is widely accepted that the views expressed in the pages of the journal were the personal views of Mrs Fenwick. Larsson probably had access to the journal when in Norway but definitely read it when she was in Edinburgh. The journal had an international distribution as the official journal of the ICN and it was read by the leaders of the nursing profession in all those countries where trained nurses were organizing for professional status. In the period 1909–11, the journal presented several articles about women's progress and kept readers updated on suffrage and women's matters.[8] Mrs Fenwick's close attention to American nursing was also reflected here.[9] In the same period, the *BJN* carried many articles and reports from the congress of the ICN that had been held in London in July 1909.[10] There were accounts of the representatives from the Nordic countries, and references to Swedish and Finnish nursing periodicals;[11] the forthcoming congress in Cologne 1912 was also discussed.[12] In 1910 articles were published written by the two Scandinavian nursing leaders, Henny Tsherning from Denmark and Sophie Mannerheim from Finland; they discussed the development of nursing in their own countries.[13]

As a significant forum for forming and exchanging views, the journal helped bring nurses together as a self-aware, nascent professionalizing group. It made the nursing world smaller and, through its pages, Larsson was able to follow international developments within the women's movement as well as in nursing.

THE CAMPAIGN FOR STATE REGISTRATION

The focus of discussion now moves to the issues dominating the nursing agenda when Larsson was in Edinburgh. The most important debates and discussions regarding state registration were pursued both in England and in Edinburgh. Accordingly, Larsson was close to the ongoing debates and the issues were familiar to her. Leading nurses and doctors working in the larger hospitals in Glasgow and Edinburgh agreed that state registration was not only desirable but also unavoidable.[14] However, they were divided as to whether Scotland should have a separate register or should share common legislation with England and Ireland. This disagreement led to the establishment of two different organizations in the Scottish campaign for state registration: the 'Scottish Nursing Association',[15] which supported common legislation with England and a single register; and the 'Association for the Registration of Nurses in Scotland', which supported separate registration for Scotland. One of the driving forces in the campaign was Lady Superintendent Miss Annie Gill. A decision to promote a common bill of registration was made by the different groups in England in 1909 and, in response, the supporters of a common system of registration between England and Scotland formed the 'Scottish Nursing Association'.[16] Miss Gill appealed for the support of all nurses for this new association,[17] a move that would unite the majority of Scottish nurses with the English groups working for state registration. Miss Gill and the nurses at the Royal Infirmary of Edinburgh joined with the majority of Scottish nurses. In addition to all the public debates and newspaper articles,[18] the close living conditions of nurses in hospitals at this time, with shared sitting rooms and dining rooms in the nurses' home, encouraged free and informal discussion of professional and private concerns.

As a leader of the national campaign for state registration, Mrs Bedford Fenwick dominated the discussions on several levels. Special attention was given to the two main reasons she advanced in support of professional independence for nursing. First, she argued that nurses and patients had to be protected from those who called themselves nurses yet had no professional education. Her second concern was the exploitation of private nurses by employers. The Registration bills that she supported incorporated three key principles. These were:

1 nurses should receive a minimum of three years' education;
2 there should be a uniform curriculum and examinations for all nurses;
3 a central nursing council should be appointed to manage the profession.[19]

Taken together, these principles promoted nursing as a distinct profession with an independent knowledge base that informed practice. They articulated and also helped sustain a vision of nursing that made it a vital part of the process of modernization taking place at that time in the healthcare system.

Private nursing and education were thoroughly discussed in the pages of the *BJN* and between 1909 and 1911 these themes received considerable attention. Much effort was made to describe the challenges that private nurses had to face on all levels and the dilemmas they encountered as professional helpers in private homes were discussed. The conclusion was that private nurses more than any other nurses needed a professional qualification.[20] One of Mrs Fenwick's arguments for state registration was precisely to protect the public from untrained private nurses, whose knowledge and personal character could be highly questionable.[21]

As to education, Mrs Fenwick, as editor, drew attention to both form and content. She also maintained that it was desirable to stress the development of a self-confident nursing character and to encourage the development of educational leadership among senior members of the profession. She also introduced debate about the role and skills of nurses for social work, and the preparation of nurse teachers as important issues. Moreover, it was claimed that those who wanted to work as midwives or psychiatric nurses should take a special education after they had finished their basic nursing education. Regarding the education of nurse teachers, Nutting's 'Teachers College' in the USA was pointed out as an exemplar for British nursing.[22]

The campaign for state registration in Britain reflected a wish to strengthen the position of nursing in society, both culturally and economically. The need for education and demarcation was legitimated in the name of the patient and in the interests of society. The arguments also reflected social ambitions. Larsson's contacts with the literature and the organizers of the campaign influenced her view of nursing as a 'bourgeois project', with culture and education as key concepts. The discussions about the campaign for state registration were a rich source of ideas and inspiration, and of great significance for Larsson's future work. After Larsson returned to Norway, her priorities reflected the professional ideas that were circulating among the pro-registration nurses in Britain at this time.

IDEALS AND IDEAS

The context of which Larsson was part in Edinburgh was one in which the women's movement was highly visible and its significance to nursing appeared obvious. A growing vision of 'women' associated inherent womanly qualities with the qualities demanded of nurses. However, to strengthen their status and position, modern professional nurses also had to dedicate themselves to progress and education based on scientific knowledge. Two fundamental and in many ways contradictory visions, therefore, challenged the development of nursing. This dual challenge was also reflected in the practical context. During her time as a nurse in Edinburgh, Larsson was immersed in the world of modernizing hospitals that attempted to unite traditional values with a belief in scientific progress.

In their practical work, nurses had to embrace new thoughts, to gain scientific knowledge and to achieve a new state of professional readiness in relation to wider changes likely to affect them and their future work. At the same time, they were also required to remain true to traditional nursing and womanly values. In this traditional aspect, their role was to draw upon and perfect their gentle inner qualities, rather than to become active agents of external change. This complex and sometimes contradictory collection of values and influences made Larsson's experience of Edinburgh nursing culture both complicated and ambiguous at the level of her personal experience.

Life on the wards at the City Hospital and the Royal Infirmary was controlled through a strict code of behaviour, in which rules required obedience, sobriety and self-sacrifice. Traditional values concerning a woman's role and appropriate religious behaviour were to be demonstrated in nurses' outward appearance and conduct.[23] In this sense, a nurse's work was grounded in personal qualities, morality and the need to follow rules governing all aspects of personal conduct and appearance. On a theoretical level, both as a nurse lecturer and in public meetings, Miss Gill expressed similar attitudes, advocating qualities such as obedience, subordination and self-sacrifice.[24] However, in her position as Lady Superintendent at the Royal Infirmary, she seemed to act in a more 'masculine' way, executing her commitments with great autonomy and authority.[25] In spite of this, she encouraged nurses to be devoted and humble, and stressed accepted womanly qualities. The values supported in this pattern of education did not encourage nurses to become sensitive or attentive to their external circumstances.

The impact of scientific knowledge upon medicine, surgery, life and death was growing at this time. This gave both the relevant knowledge, and those who laid claim to it, a special position and status. This scientific medical knowledge was primarily the property of doctors. However, the rapid growth of healthcare provision in the early twentieth century required doctors to share their scientific knowledge with nurses, at least to a degree. This gave nurses a potentially more significant role. Paradoxically, it made them both more independent of, and also more dependent on, the doctors. Access to medical knowledge became a means of raising the status of nurses, and it gave them the opportunity to develop their role within a professionalizing healthcare system. The combination of scientific knowledge with the womanly qualities emphasized in traditional nursing culture had the potential to make nurses significant actors in the modernization process of medicine. This was the world into which Larsson arrived at the Royal Infirmary of Edinburgh in 1909.

Larsson was able to study nursing education at first hand at the Royal Infirmary, one of the most prestigious and largest hospitals in Great Britain, and this served as an example for her. The school of nursing was a well-established Nightingale-inspired institution that had long offered a three-year training course. The Lady Superintendent led the education and, as such, Miss Gill became Larsson's role model. Larsson would have been aware that Miss Gill was fighting to extend the nursing training from three to four years (she succeeded in 1911). In addition, she observed the range of different courses provided for trained nurses enabling them to consolidate their knowledge in physiology, hygiene and nutrition.

We know, therefore, that Larsson was exposed to a range of ideals and ideas on several levels during her time in Edinburgh. These demonstrated how women introduced and promoted significant social change, both individually and in groups across several nursing and non-nursing contexts. In Edinburgh, she found nursing delicately poised between innovations promoting new forms of organization, expertise, knowledge and professionalism, and the support of traditional appeals to a vocational inner calling that valued female qualities that were assumed to be socially immutable.

RETURNING TO NORWAY

Coming back to Norway in 1911, Larsson started to work as a private nurse in Kristiania. This gave her first-hand knowledge of working conditions in this field and can be interpreted as a strategic move, influenced by the impressions she had formed about private nursing during her stay in Scotland. The conditions within the private nursing field made it a weak link in the process of professionalization. Through her articles in the *BJN*, Mrs Fenwick had contributed to the view that regarded private nurses as an obstacle to nursing reform. According to Larsson, the conditions in private nursing in Kristiania were bad. She claimed that it was far too easy to be engaged as a private nurse; as a result unsuitable women were recruited and employed as private nurses.[26]

At the beginning of the twentieth century, the number of secular nurses in Norway was increasing and it was this expansion in numbers that constituted the basis for the founding of a national nursing association. Besides, organizing such groupings was a common feature at the time.[27] In 1911 the nurses' conditions of work were still unstandardized and the nurse training schools, the numbers of which were growing, were characterized by their variation in both the duration and the contents of the education and training that they offered. Secular nurses were particularly disadvantaged as, unlike the deaconesses, they had no 'mother-house' that could provide for their future security. This was a powerful argument for the founding of a national professional organization.

WORK OF PREPARATION

After a year as a private nurse, Larsson began the final preparatory work that was to lead to the formation of a national nursing association in Norway. In the spring of 1912, she wrote to Henny Tscherning, leader of the Danish Nursing Association. She requested information about the establishment of the Danish Association, the Danish periodical, *Sygeplejersken,* and nursing education in Denmark. Later she also wrote to Sophie Mannerheim in Finland and obtained similar information from her. At the same time, she made contact with the Norwegian Council of Women (NCW). In an interview in their periodical, *Nylænde*, Larsson introduced many of the themes that had appeared in the *British Journal of Nursing* while she was in Edinburgh. There is other evidence that indicates increasing contact between Larsson and the leader of the NCW, Gina Krog, in the year 1912. Before this date *Nylænde* had paid scant attention to nurses and their position. From 1912, articles about nurses and nursing began to appear in the periodical. These included an article that discussed the establishment of the NNA.[28] Larsson also established contact with the Norwegian Medical Association (NMA) and received a range of advice about how to prepare for the foundation of a professional association.[29] It is worth pausing to consider why Larsson wanted to make the NCW and the NMA her allies.

First of all, Gina Krog and the Norwegian Council of Women had supported the establishment of several trade unions for women. In addition, the NCW had a strong public position and their support would be of great value to a nursing association. The members of the NCW were, like Larsson herself, mainly unmarried women from the middle class. Accordingly, a closer connection between the two organizations was likely to make nursing more attractive to middle-class women. Entering into an alliance with the NCW therefore had the potential to strengthen the status of Norwegian nursing. This alliance between the NCW and the NNA followed an international tradition of strong ties between nursing associations and the women's movement. This proved to be a worthwhile connection; Gina Krog and the NCW gave Larsson significant support before, during and after the founding of the NNA.

Establishing contact with the Norwegian Medical Association was both a strategic and a necessary move. This initiative of Larsson's reflected her conclusion that not only did the doctors need skilled nurses, but also that skilled nurses needed the doctors. In her view, getting in touch with the NMA promoted good will towards the foundation of a nursing association, and therefore formed a valuable starting point for future cooperation between the two professions. Second, the doctors were key figures in the improvement of nursing education. They were both guardians and teachers of the knowledge through which skilled nursing might strengthen its status and position. Continuing developments within the field of medicine constituted another important reason for entering into a closer relationship with the medical profession. A developing relationship with the NMA would give nurses access to new areas of knowledge and legitimate their need for theoretical education. An alliance with the medical profession would serve several purposes, and be of great significance for the strengthening of the status and position of nursing.

In the summer of 1912, Larsson travelled to Denmark and Germany.[30] In Copenhagen she met Henny Tscherning; Mrs Tscherning had studied nursing both at the Royal Infirmary of Edinburgh and at St Thomas' Hospital in London, and was an internationally acknowledged nursing leader. As a leader of the Danish Nursing Association, she worked for a standardized three-year nursing education and state registration.[31] In Denmark and Norway, nurses faced similar problems regarding education and working conditions. Larsson met members of the German Nursing Association and obtained information regarding its establishment. The German Association was well connected to both the ICN and the ICW. Almost single-handedly the energetic leader of the German Nursing Association, Agnes Karll, had placed education, working conditions and the rights of German nurses on the national agenda.[32] It is clear that there were common features for Danish, German and British nursing; these included the struggle for improvement of working conditions and education, and for state registration. Similarly, the secular nurses in these countries had their own national associations with links to both the ICN and the ICW.

In August 1912, Larsson, together with four other Norwegian nurses, attended her first ICN congress in Cologne. The main subjects on the programme were education, the development of nursing as a profession, and finally the extension of women's rights.[33] Larsson later expressed great enthusiasm for the Congress, which gave her the opportunity to meet the most significant women in nursing at the time: Agnes Karll, Adelaide Nutting, Lillian Wald, Ethel Bedford Fenwick and Lavinia Lloyd Dock. As a cadre they had much in common: they came from wealthy families and held important national positions in nursing; they were closely involved with the women's movement and were fighting for female rights; and they regarded the conditions of nursing and women's rights as part of the same agenda. The subjects that dominated the ICN programme, women's rights, the public role of women, the position and status of nursing, education, and competent and incompetent nursing, confirmed the importance of the issues that Larsson had observed during her years in Edinburgh.

The letters Larsson wrote to prominent nursing leaders in Scandinavia, as well as the trips she made in the summer of 1912, indicate that she acted in a definite way to obtain information about the organization of nursing in other countries. They also indicate that there was communication and an exchange of ideas between nurses at an international level. In Cologne she became further aware of the importance of establishing a nursing association in Norway and of the advantages of a broader international participation. The congress contributed to her vision and provided her with inspiration. The form it took, as well as the content of the debates, created a dynamic picture of nurses; by combining female qualities and modern scientific education nurses had the opportunity to form a profession with great significance for the development of society.

THE FOUNDING OF THE NORWEGIAN NURSING ASSOCIATION

The Norwegian Nursing Association (NNA) was established on 24 September 1912, shortly after the congress in Cologne. Larsson had made all the preparations, including drafting the rules and regulations, in advance of this first meeting, and the forty-four nurses personally selected by Larsson to attend applauded and unanimously approved her initiative. Larsson was elected leader, a position she held until 1935. It can be argued that the founding of the NNA gave Larsson the opportunity to address two areas that had been much debated while she was abroad: women's qualities and their education. These areas were given prominence throughout the period she was President of the organization.

The new association was welcomed by the international nursing world. Larsson received congratulatory telegrams from Germany, England, Denmark, Finland and Sweden, and Lavinia Dock sent good wishes from the USA. Shortly after the NNA was established, the first issue of the periodical *Sykepleien* appeared, with Larsson as editor. The newly elected leader of the NNA gave private nursing priority, and in particular the distinction between 'suitable women' and those considered 'unsuitable'.

Larsson's purpose to divide 'suitable' nurses from those considered 'unsuitable' was reflected in her choice of the forty-four nurses who attended the founding meeting. They were primarily women who earned their own living through paid work and they reflected a trend among unmarried middle-class women. Like Larsson, most of them were well educated for their time; many of them had studied nursing abroad and several had good positions in hospitals and were considered pioneers in Norwegian nursing. In effect, Larsson had invited women who represented a kind of 'elite' among Norwegian nurses. Most of the forty-four nurses came from Kristiania and from the larger cities in Norway. They set up a standard for the new association and showed the outside world who the skilled nurses were and with whom they wished to be identified. The choice of the forty-four elite nurses indicates that a strong driving force in Larsson's project from the beginning was to associate nursing with socially elevated groups.

Similar ambitions were reflected in the rules and regulations for membership of the NNA.[34] To be a member of the organization, a certain level of education was required and, in effect, Larsson used the regulations for membership to define who had the right to call themselves nurses. For these members she recommended uniforms, badges and clearly written rules of conduct; the assumption was that by their appearance and behaviour nurses should be exemplary women. Further, the regulations proposed how others should perceive skilled nurses both ethically and aesthetically. Finally, they also encouraged a sense of identity among nurses themselves. As discussed earlier in this chapter, this was very similar to attitudes promoted within the practice settings of the Edinburgh hospitals where she had worked. Such requirements were primarily directed towards personal morality and the perfection of inner character, rather than outwards to the wider political, economic and social contexts within which nurses worked. At the ICN congress in Cologne similar values had been stressed; professional nursing had to be based on education, high moral standards and suitability. The NNA took the international position seriously from the very beginning. The stand against unskilled nurses was to be pursued.

Private nursing received Larsson's immediate attention; she fought considerable battles with the authorities to achieve regulation of nurses working in the private sphere. The arguments she used were the same as those put forward about private nursing in the *British Journal of Nursing*; patients had to be protected from unskilled nurses and from the potential danger they represented.[35] As in England and Scotland, the majority of private nurses in Norway were unskilled nurses recruited from the lower classes in society. This was damaging to the image of nursing. As a group, the unskilled private nurses represented a threat to all the values and goals promoted by the international nursing organization. One-and-a-half years after its foundation, the NNA was permitted to run an employment agency by the Norwegian authorities.[36] The establishment of this special nursing bureau made it possible for the NNA to check the credentials of nurses and to recommend skilled nurses to the public; only nurses satisfying the regulations of the NNA were employed. This was an important step towards professional control of nursing and also towards the state registration of practitioners.

Nursing education in general became Larsson's main concern. She adopted the key principles of a minimum three-year training course, a uniform curriculum and examinations for all nurses; education, she argued, would divide 'suitable' from 'unsuitable women'. Still she hesitated to put the principle of a three-year training programme on NNA's formal agenda. Why was this so? In Norway the supply of skilled nurses was small; further, the quality of nurse education was very variable and few nurses had pedagogical skills. As a result, few nurses were competent to become teachers of nursing and to supervise nursing students. Larsson attempted to resolve this problem by introducing schemes aimed at furthering the competence of the existing trained nurses. She encouraged nurses to take advanced studies in nursing. Major efforts were made to help nurses improve education in the larger hospitals. She was also eager to send educated nurses abroad, to help them develop their skills in supervising nursing students in the wards. She was prepared to use money and also her personal influence to establish such arrangements. The letters to Larsson from Annie Gill, Lady Superintendent at the Royal Infirmary of Edinburgh, provide one example of this strategy at work during 1913; several Norwegian nursing students went to Edinburgh to study nursing on the recommendation of Larsson.[37]

Strengthening the competence of skilled nurses in Norway was undoubtedly a matter of great importance for Larsson, and probably the main reason why she postponed the question of a uniform three-year training course. Instead it was the doctors who put the issue on the formal agenda in 1915. A committee consisting of six nurses, among them Larsson, eight doctors and two ministers were selected to prepare a bill to prescribe the education of nurses. However, they could not reach agreement about the duration of the nurses' education. The majority suggested two different courses, one of eighteen months duration, the other of three years duration. The minority, including Larsson and another pioneer nurse in Norway, Andrea Arntzen, would not accept anything but a uniform three-year training course. When the medical association suggested promoting the majority's proposal to the government, Larsson composed a letter recommending the postponement of a decision; 650 nurses and eighty-five doctors signed this letter. She claimed that, until a sufficient number of three-year training courses had been established in Norway, a postponement of the bill was in the nurses' best interests. She also maintained that, to her, the idea of an eighteen-month education for district nurses was both strange and extremely unfavourable for the development of nursing. Like private nurses, district nurses held independent positions in nursing and in her opinion their need of a three-year education was obvious.

Why did Larsson fight so hard to avoid two different kinds of training courses for nurses? A uniform education of three years duration was intended to raise the level of knowledge in nursing and to provide an equal standard among nurses. One of the aims of this policy was to strengthen the social position and status of nurses, and to ensure the conditions for further professionalization. This would make nursing more attractive to middle-class women. In addition, a uniform education and also registration were considered very important for international mobility and migration. The international nursing leaders claimed that to internationalize nursing, it first had to be standardized.[38] Consequently, two different training courses represented a threat to the ambitions Larsson had on behalf of Norwegian nursing. To her great satisfaction, she succeeded in delaying the issue for nearly ten years.

In the mean time, Larsson implemented several initiatives to achieve her goals. In 1917, together with her colleague Andrea Arntzen, she designed a curriculum for a three-year training course. This was very similar to the one at the Royal Infirmary of Edinburgh. The NNA published the curriculum as an example for nursing education in Norway. Only those schools that introduced the curriculum were approved and recognized as providing a full education by the NNA. In this way, the NNA started its own authorization of nursing courses. In 1921 the regulations for membership of the organization were altered. Despite considerable opposition, especially from the doctors, a three-year training course in nursing was required to qualify as a member of the NNA.[39] In a short time, the number of three-year training courses increased dramatically in Norway.

In 1925 Larsson took the initiative to establish courses for qualified nurses. The example she used was provided by Bedford College in London. From 1920 Bedford College had offered an international one-year nursing course in administration, teaching and social work. The Norwegian courses were named 'Norwegian Nurses courses for superior and teaching nurses, together with social workers'.[40] The content of the courses shows the inclusion of scientific knowledge with womanly qualities, but also masculine strategies, all were considered to be essential. Larsson argued that nurses, to be able to participate in the same way as men in society, had to learn about politics and legislation. They also had to learn how to make a speech and how to argue in public. In this way, Norwegian nurses would strengthen their competence and be prepared to take leading positions on several levels within different areas in society.[41] During the first ten years, approximately 300 nurses undertook the courses arranged by Larsson and the NNA.[42] Not only Norwegian nurses, but nurses from the whole of Scandinavia enrolled on the courses.

During the 1920s much effort was made to improve the conditions in Norwegian nursing education. At the beginning of 1930s, the medical profession changed its opinion and decided to support the nurses in their claim for a uniform three-year training course and state registration. Despite this, a final resolution concerning state registration was not made until 1948.

At the beginning of 1930s, Larsson gradually began to lose her position as leader of the NNA. Changing times had brought new ideas, values and attitudes that had influenced nurses and they made new demands on their leader. Larsson was challenged by the members and was particularly criticized for giving too much importance and resources to education and international nursing. As a result, they claimed, too little attention was given to the problems Norwegian nurses experienced in their work situations. In 1935 Larsson resigned her position as leader of the NNA. The new demands of the membership were not compatible with her long-standing ideas.

CONCLUSION

Bergljot Larsson was a resourceful and energetic person; her decision at the age of twenty-six years 'to study nursing' abroad in 1909, is testimony to that. Edinburgh and Great Britain were significant and dynamic places for her development as both a woman and a nurse, and they contributed significantly to what was a 'defining moment' in her career. Her experience in Edinburgh supported and nourished her growing ideas about women and nursing. She was confirmed in her view of women as significant contributors to the process of creating a better society, and nurses as significant contributors to the modernization process in early twentieth-century health services.

Her views of the women's movement, and its interconnections with nursing, were strengthened through Mrs Fenwick and her *British Journal of Nursing* and by the exemplary Miss Gill, both of whom were leaders involved with the campaign for state registration in Britain. Her views received further confirmation through the ICN congress in Cologne. The congress must be looked upon as a definitive source of inspiration for Larsson. Here she renewed existing contacts and met new nurse leaders. The contacts she made with Scandinavian and German nursing after returning to Norway gave her practical insights and the information that enabled her to transform her vision for Norwegian nursing into the practical reality of the NNA.

Larsson's belief in the potential and significance of women's special qualities, combined with modern nursing education, were reflected in the alliances she established and the priorities she set as a leader of the NNA. The foundation of the NNA was the most important enterprise she engaged in; it was a crucial strategy that allowed Larsson to achieve the objectives she had formulated while abroad.

By way of conclusion, we can reflect more generally upon Larsson's international contacts and their influence upon her work. It can be claimed that she was more concerned to implement existing ideas and motivations than to become an innovative, original and freethinking nurse in her own right. The establishment of the NNA was a pioneering act in national terms but its inspiration was firmly rooted in international nursing developments.

NOTES

1   Minute-book, Kristiania Municipal Hospital 1903–1920. The archive of Ullevål Hospital.
2   Minute-book, Kristiania Municipal Nursing Association, 1907–1919. The archive of the Norwegian Nursing Association (NNA).
3   S. Hvalvik, "'Elever modtages til oplærelse i Sygepleien' En historisk analyse av sykepleieutdanningens framvekst i Telemark perioden 1890–1919", hovedfagsoppgave, Institutt for Sykepleievitenskap, Universitetet i Oslo, Oslo. 1996.
4   Reference signed by J. Thomas, Matron, at the City Hospital, Comiston Road, Edinburgh, 19 May 1910. Certified copy from Records, signed by E. D. Smaill, Lady Superintendent of Nurses, Edinburgh 6 June 1935. Private sources.
5   M. Vicinius, *Independent Women: Work and Community for Single Women 1850–1920*, London: Virago Press, 1985, pp. 252–80.
6   E. Thomson, 'Women in medicine in late nineteenth and early twentieth century Edinburgh: a case study', unpublished PhD thesis, University of Edinburgh. 1998, p. 74.
7   D. C. Bridges, *A History of the International Council of Nurses 1899–1964*, London: Pitman Medical Publishing, 1967.
8   'Nurses national journals', *British Journal of Nursing*, 1910, Vol. 44, pp. 54–5; 'Medical women and the suffrage', *British Journal of Nursing*, 1910, Vol. 44, p. 175; 'Outside the gates: women', *British Journal of Nursing*, 1910, Vol. 44, p. 56; 'Outside the gates: women [Lady Constance Lytton and Mrs Pethick Lawrence]', *British Journal of Nursing*, 1910, Vol. 44, p. 95.
9   'The central preparatory course for nurses at Teachers College, New York', *British Journal of Nursing*, 1910, Vol. 44, p. 47; 'Professional review: visiting nursing in the United States', *British Journal of Nursing*, 1910, Vol. 44, pp. 55–6; 'A hospital to teach straight thinking [New York]', *British Journal of Nursing*, 1910, Vol. 44, pp. 92–3; 'Letter from Miss Nutting', *British Journal of Nursing*, 1910, Vol. 44, p. 95; 'State registration in the United States', *British Journal of Nursing*, 1910, Vol. 44, p. 106; L. L. Dock, 'Our foreign letter: from the United States', *British Journal of Nursing*, 1910, Vol. 44, pp. 479–80.

10 B. Kent, 'The nurse in private practice (read at the International Congress of Nurses, London, July 1909)', *British Journal of Nursing,* 1910, Vol. 44, pp. 3–4 and 23–4; A. Salvador, 'The nurse in private practice (read at the International Congress of Nurses, London, July 1909)', *British Journal of Nursing,* 1910, Vol. 44, pp. 45–6; E. Schopwinkel, 'Private nursing in Germany' (read at the International Congress of Nurses, London, July 1909)', *British Journal of Nursing,* 1910, Vol. 44, pp. 64–5; J. C. van Lanschot-Hubrecht, 'A special curriculum for private nurses (read at the International Congress of Nurses, London, July 1909)', *British Journal of Nursing,* 1910, Vol. 44, pp. 83–4; E. M. Musson, 'Hospital kitchens (read at the International Congress of Nurses, London, July 1909)', *British Journal of Nursing,* 1910, Vol. 44, pp. 107–9.

11 'International news', *British Journal of Nursing,* 1910, Vol. 44, p. 28; 'State registration in Finland', *British Journal of Nursing,* 1910, Vol. 44, pp. 129–30; 'Swedish Nurses Association', *British Journal of Nursing,* 1910, Vol. 44, p. 325.

12 'The Cologne Congress', *British Journal of Nursing,* 1910, Vol. 44, p. 78; 'The Cologne Congress', *British Journal of Nursing,* 1910, Vol. 44, p. 98.

13 H. Tscherning, 'The Danish Council of Nurses', *British Journal of Nursing,* 1910, Vol. 44, p. 15; 'International news', *British Journal of Nursing,* 1910, Vol. 44, p. 28.

14 *British Journal of Nursing,* 1909, Vol. 42 p. 147.

15 'The Scottish Nurses Association', *British Journal of Nursing,* 1910, Vol. 44, pp. 248–9.

16 'Association for the Promotion of Registration of Nurses in Scotland', *British Journal of Nursing,* 1910, Vol. 44, pp. 207–8.

17 *British Journal of Nursing,* 1911, Vol. 46, pp. 168–9.

18 Ibid., Mrs Fenwick acknowledged the *Scotsman* as a source for her article.

19 S. McGann, *The Battle of the Nurses: A Study of Eight Women who Influenced the Development of Professional Nursing, 1880–1930,* London: Scutari Press, 1992.

20 *British Journal of Nursing,* 1910, Vol. 44, pp. 3, 24, 45, 64, 83.

21 *British Journal of Nursing,* 1910, Vol. 45, p. 527.

22 *British Journal of Nursing,* 1911, Vol. 47, p. 81.

23 Edinburgh City Hospital, 'Nursing Staff Regulations'; The Royal Infirmary, Edinburgh. 'Regulations as to uniform', Private sources. Lothian Health Service Archive (LHSA) LHB1/5/14, 'Rules and Regulations of the RIE', Special Collections, University of Edinburgh.

24 LHSA, MAC GD1/39, Nursing Lectures: Notes from Miss Gill's lecture, 13 October 1910, "Nursing ethics and hospital etiquette"; MAC GD1/22, Nursing Lectures: Notes from Miss Gill's lecture, 20 October 1910, "A nurse's duty to herself".

25 LHSA, LHB1/2/54, 'Minute Book of Nursing Committee, 1909–1911'.

26 *Sykepleien,* 1913, Vol. 1, no. 4, p. 35.

27 K. Melby, *Kall og Kamp: Norsk Sykepleierforbunds historie,* Oslo: Cappelen, 1990, p. 41.

28 *Nylænde,* 1912, Vol. 26, p. 342

29 *Sykepleien,* 1912, Vol. 1, no. 1, p. 7.

30 *Sykepleien,* 1913, Vol. 1, p. 80.

31 E. Petersen, *Sygeplejesagens pioner, Henny Tscherning 1853–1932,* København: Dansk Sygeplejeråd, 1998.

32 G. Boschma, 'Agnes Karll and the creation of an independent nursing association 1900–1927', *Nursing History Review,* 1996, Vol. 4, pp. 151–168.

33 Bridges, *History of the International Council of Nurses.*

34 The Norwegian Nursing Association 1912–1962, NNA Archives.

35 *Sykepleien,* 1913, Vol. 1, pp. 80–1.

36 *Sykepleien,* 1914, Vol. 2, no. 2, p. 20.

37   Letter to Bergljot Larsson from Miss Annie Gill, 21 November 1913, NNA Archives.
38   A. M. Rafferty, and G. Boschma, 'The essential idea', in: B. L. Brush and J. Lynaugh (eds), *Nurses of all Nations, a History of the International Council of Nurses, 1899–1999,* Philadelphia: Lippincott, 1999, p. 53.
39   *Sykepleien,* 1922, Vol. 10, no. 1, p. 7.
40   *Sykepleien,* 1925, Vol. 13, no. 9, p. 63.
41   *Politics of Women,* Larsson 5. NNA archives.
42   Sykepleien, 1937, Vol. 25, no. 9. p. 126.

4 Puerperal fever as a source of conflict between midwives and medical men in eighteenth- and early nineteenth-century Britain

Christine E. Hallett

The idea that midwives and medical men fought for control of childbirth in the eighteenth century has long been viewed as a part of the history of midwifery. It is an idea that has been accepted implicitly by most writers on the subject, even those who have warned that it might be an over-simplification.[1] Originating from very different social backgrounds, the two groups operated from within radically different knowledge bases and drew on unique bodies of experience that overlapped less than might be supposed.

MIDWIFERY PRACTICE IN THE EIGHTEENTH AND EARLY NINETEENTH CENTURIES

Traditional midwifery had a long and established record of providing care and service to women in childbirth. Midwives were placed within a recognized and defined social role, which was sanctioned and controlled by local powers, both secular and religious; powers that recognized and accepted norms of apprenticeship-style training.

'Medical men', as I refer to them here, were an apparently inchoate group who shared certain important features that distinguished them from traditional midwives. All these men had some formal education and training. Physicians, who held the qualification MD, had been awarded a university degree, whereas surgeons' skills were recognized by guild or corporation membership. In addition to their status as members of recognized and formally educated groups, physicians and surgeons were usually drawn from gentry backgrounds, and were always men. The traditional midwives were women from lower social orders, with little or no formal education. In many ways the two groups could not have been more socially distinct.[2]

The superior learning and education of medical men had evolved over time. Until the mid-eighteenth century, the practice of surgeons had been regulated by guilds and was closely associated with barbers. In London, the Barber-Surgeons Company (established by Act of Parliament in 1540) was the significant regulatory body for surgical practice until 1745, when the Company of Surgeons split from the barber-surgeons. During the second half of the eighteenth century, a new form of practitioner, the surgeon-apothecary, became increasingly important. In addition to completing several years surgical apprenticeship, these practitioners had often acquired knowledge and education by attending private anatomy schools; one of the most famous of these schools had been established in Great Windmill Street, London, by William Hunter in 1770. Some surgeon-apothecaries also attended courses at university medical schools, sometimes travelling abroad to centres of excellence, for example to Paris or Leiden, to extend both their education and their practical experience.[3]

The term 'general-practitioner' had emerged by the end of the eighteenth century. These practitioners were highly educated and experienced individuals, who often held licences from both the Royal College of Surgeons and the Society of Apothecaries; many also held university medical degrees. The Apothecaries Act, passed in 1815, regulated this group.[4] In the course of the eighteenth century, the term 'man-midwife' was increasingly used to refer to male practitioners of midwifery, many of whom also adopted the French term 'accoucheur', perhaps to avoid the gender anomaly implicit in the British term.[5]

Physicians formed the most elite group among the male practitioners and were required to hold a university degree in medicine. Their area of special expertise had always been accepted as 'internal medicine,' a term that distinguished their practice from the work of surgeons on the 'external' structure of the body. The majority of practitioners who wrote on subjects such as puerperal fever – and certainly most of those who are cited in this chapter – held a degree, mostly obtained from those universities that were regarded as the most dynamic and effective in the eighteenth and early nineteenth centuries, that is Edinburgh, Leiden and, to a lesser extent, Paris.[6]

The traditional midwives were a more complicated group than first appearances suggest. The majority of those individuals who referred to themselves as 'midwives' were trained through apprenticeship; they were licensed by religious and/or secular authorities and they practised only midwifery. There was, however, an important 'overlap' between this group and women described as 'nurses', a complex and largely unregulated group who practised in a wide range of social settings. It is likely that some nurses, particularly those working in rural areas, also practised midwifery. There were also women who specialized in the work of caring for mothers and babies during the first month after delivery, who were often referred to as 'monthly nurses'.

The involvement of these distinct groups of practitioners in childbirth, and the complications of birthing, had important consequences. Prior to the mid-eighteenth century, it had been usual for the care of women in childbirth to be the joint work of midwives and surgeons. Midwives, with the help of the childbearing woman's female relatives and friends, took care of normal labours and deliveries. Surgeons were called in only to deal with abnormal or problematic births, and then often only when a child was already dead and needed to be extracted from the womb to save the mother's life. This system appeared to work relatively well for the practitioners involved. It did, however, exclude physicians. This meant, as a number of writers have commented, that normal childbirth was assisted, surrounded and almost 'hedged in' by female traditional knowledge in a way that, to the men of the early modern period, must have appeared deliberately to exclude them from any real involvement.[7]

THE MEDICAL WRITINGS OF THE EIGHTEENTH AND EARLY NINETEENTH CENTURIES

It has already been suggested that to view the eighteenth century as a period in which medical men wrested control of childbirth from traditional midwives is to over-simplify a complex reality. It is, nevertheless, indisputably the case that many more 'normal', uncomplicated labours and deliveries were managed by medical practitioners by the end of the century than at the start.[8] If it is appropriate to regard midwives and medical men as engaged in some kind of dispute or war for the control of childbirth, one significant area – one of their battlegrounds – was that of puerperal fever. This was a battleground where the medical men were always at an advantage and where the midwives were always obliged to adopt a defensive position, for it involved a subject – fever – over which medicine had always claimed expert knowledge. Essentially, medical men claimed the possession of superior knowledge and expertise, a claim that could be justified as the eighteenth century moved on if the expansion of their midwifery practice among wealthy clients is accepted as evidence of success. Claims to superiority by medical men had important consequences, and they raise questions that are of enduring importance in any examination of the relationship between groups of practitioners. Three of these questions will be examined here. First, what does it mean when a discipline declares itself to be more scientific than competing disciplines? Second, what is the purpose of such a claim? Third, to what extent does the claim impact upon the interests of the patient?

In the 1770s, Charles White, the Manchester-based physician and man-midwife, described the nurses of London as a 'numerous and powerful body'. Presumably he was referring to the monthly nurses who took care of women in the lying-in period after delivery. He stated: 'The articles of air, diet, dress, etc. are left to the management of nurses in that city, who claim it as a kind of prerogative, and it is next to sacrilege to encroach upon their privileges.'[9]

White's claim might have a rhetorical element to it. Nevertheless, he appears to express genuine concern. He certainly represented the nurses as a group powerful enough to undermine the work of the physician. He went on to discuss how difficult it is for his colleagues to overcome this problem:

> A young man just coming into business might justly think it too daring an attempt to encounter them; he would in all probability be unequal to the task, and his future progress would be stopped by making such powerful enemies. The man in full and established business could not perhaps spare so much time as would be necessary, for it would require a very frequent and constant attendance upon his patients to see that the nurses did their duty; and by such an attempt he might lose much and gain little, except trouble and opposition.[10]

Here we find an eighteenth-century medical practitioner referring repeatedly to the power of the nurses in a way that is most intriguing. Wherein does their power lie? It appears to have its basis in the constancy of the nurse's presence at the bedside. The physician might have a monopoly of the giving of 'medical' advice, but the nurse has the power to implement or ignore his instructions. At first sight this would seem to set narrow boundaries to her authority. But a crucial element in the power structure was, of course, the patient's willingness to comply with the physician's regimen. Very often in the medical treatises referred to in this chapter there is a suggestion of confederacy between nurse and patient, who might make a joint decision to ignore medical instructions.

A marked characteristic of the writings of physicians on the subject of child-birth was their tendency to be critical of existing traditional or lay knowledge in the field. Numerous examples of work from this period can be interpreted as characteristic of an effort to broaden the power and scope of medical 'expertise'. These writings range from works on health written for the benefit of ladies[11] to works on nursing and the care of children (formerly almost exclusively female preserves)[12] and manuals of instruction for female midwives.[13] A tendency to chastise and lecture non-medical carers was a common feature of the writings of medical men during this period. The same tendency not only found its way into texts on midwifery, it was a feature of a range of mainstream texts, dealing with common and serious illnesses. For example, a work on pulmonary tuberculosis written in 1782 by Reid, a physician, criticized attempts at curing this disease with home-made remedies. He used deliberately strong and vivid language to drive home his point, referring to these non-medical remedies as 'greasy emulsions and a profusion of palling sweets'.[14] The tendency of medical treatise writers to devote so much space within their works to the criticism of approaches other than their own suggests that they believed the knowledge and expertise of their non-medical competitors to be a serious threat to their own status and practice. John Clarke observed in 1793:

> With respect to improper treatment after delivery this is partly to be imputed to the accoucheur in some instances perhaps, but much more frequently to the woman herself, either using some indulgences of the appetite, which are incompatible with her situation, or to the well-meant, but ill-judged advice of her friends, or the obstinacy of bad nurses.[15]

This phrase 'the obstinacy of bad nurses' resonates through the historical record of the eighteenth and early nineteenth centuries, but what were the actions of 'bad nurses' in this context? They might include giving spicy, strongly alcoholic caudles to lying-in women and impeding ventilation in the lying-in chamber. 'Bad nurses' might allow the patient meat instead of thin gruel, if she wished it, and permit the patient to adopt the positions she preferred rather than those dictated by the latest medical opinion that were thought to encourage drainage of the lochia or prevent the pooling of blood in the pelvis.

The obstinate bad nurses were 'unscientific' practitioners. And yet even among these supposedly uneducated individuals there were those such as Jane Sharp, Sarah Stone and Elizabeth Nihell, who wrote with intelligence and authority on a range of issues relating to childbirth.[16] The female authors were in broad agreement with the mainstream of medical writing about a range of subjects. They emphasized, in particular, the importance of avoiding undue interference in the process of childbirth and could be scathing in their criticisms of colleagues who did force the pace of a labour and delivery. They also emphasized the need for a good knowledge of the anatomy of the pelvis.[17]

MEDICAL THEORIES OF PUERPERAL FEVER

Puerperal fever posed a particularly intractable problem for both traditional and medically trained midwives in the eighteenth and nineteenth centuries. Contemporaries recognized that they had a poor understanding of this disease and there were numerous attempts to explain it with reference to prevailing scientific theories; inflammatory theory was the most prominent of these. According to this theory, fevers were the consequence of a 'lentor' or viscidity of the blood, which could be forced through the blood vessels only if the circulatory system worked much harder and more quickly than usual. This would result in a rapid pulse and a general 'excitability' of the system that, if untreated, could lead to collapse. Within the theoretical perspective of the medical men, the tendency of traditional midwives to offer women spicy, alcoholic 'caudles' and to keep them in warm, relatively airless conditions would only worsen this situation.

Some medical men, prominent among them Charles White, emphasized what they saw as the putrid nature of the disease. Some saw putrefaction as an end stage of the inflammatory process. According to this alternative account favoured by White and others, putrefaction was the central process of the disease. They linked it to inflammation but saw it rather as the cause than as the consequence of that condition. In common with the inflammationists, the putrefactionists saw overheating the patient as dangerous, as this led to the more rapid stagnation of trapped secretions – seen as the root cause of fever.

White offered an interesting narrative in his treatise of 1777. He referred to a woman who had given birth to her third child on 21 April 1770.[18] He noticed that, whenever he visited her, 'she was always in a sweat'. The room was very hot, as a large fire was kept constantly ablaze, and the air had a 'disagreeable smell'. He related that he gave instructions that the patient should be kept cool and the room well ventilated, 'but none of these directions were complied with'. He then spoke to the patient's husband about her condition, and was informed that the nurse, the child and two other women had slept in the room with the mother since her delivery, and that none of the physician's instructions had been followed:

> ... for if we opened a door, it was shut immediately after our leaving the house, that a large fire had been kept in the room day and night; that the curtains had always been drawn close round her bed, and that she had not

been permitted to breathe any air but what had been polluted by her sweat and excrements, and the effluvia arising from the breath of so many persons.[19]

The husband was now said to have realized that his wife's health was being damaged. He thus took action, stating that he 'was now sensible both of the danger she was in, and of the absurdity of the practice of those about her'. He had the fire removed and the room cooled and ventilated. In consequence, the reader is told, the patient recovered. White added that she had subsequently had another child, and that 'during her last lying-in she strictly observed the directions I gave, and had no fever or other bad symptoms.'[20]

Alongside White's narrative, it is worth considering the account of Alexander Gordon of Aberdeen. Gordon observed that, in Aberdeen, a 'very powerful prejudice prevailed' against what he viewed as the proper treatment for puerperal fever, that is bleeding and purging – regarded as suitable remedies to counteract inflammatory processes. He posited that this prejudice was due to a failure on the part of female practitioners to recognize the nature of puerperal fever. He suggested that the women viewed the fever as a variant of the ephemeral fever known as 'the weed':

> On this ground, heating cordials were profusely exhibited by female practitioners, who are as numerous now in Aberdeen as they were formerly in London in the days of Sydenham; but they obtained no great credit by such a practice, for none who were treated in this manner recovered.[21]

Gordon recounted the case of Isabel Allen, whose condition he found to have worsened on the second day of the disease, adding, 'I had not much reason to be surprised at this, as none of my orders had been obeyed. I therefore considered the case as hopeless'.[22]

A third theory, vitalism, was strongly favoured by some physicians in their attempts to understand puerperal fever. This account emphasized the importance of nervous energy and saw illness and debility as the consequence of a lack of such energy. Adherents of vitalist philosophy viewed putrefaction as an important precursor of nervous debility, which, if allowed to progress, could result in death. Along with the inflammationists and putrefactionists, the vitalists emphasized the dangers of spicy drinks and hot airless conditions.

John Armstrong, whose treatise was published in 1814, was adamant about the dangers of bad practice by midwives and monthly nurses. He commented that it was 'not uncommon' for nurses to give spicy and alcoholic caudles to lying-in women, sometimes 'expressly against the commands of medical practitioners'. He added:

> The deceptions practised by those persons commonly called old experienced nurses, are hardly credible; in the presence of the physicians, they will seem very desirous to carry all his orders into effect, but in his absence, either accommodate themselves to the whims of the capricious or, appealing to their

long experience persuade the timorous patient to take a diet very different from that directed; and thus, between the hypocrisy of the one and the weakness of the other, the deceit is successfully carried on, unless danger or accident should reveal it. The lives of many women, and the reputations of many accoucheurs have, I am fully confident, been sacrificed in this way.[23]

But not all midwives and nurses were 'obstinate'. The following extract, taken from a description by Whitehead – an adherent of putrefaction theory – of action taken during the puerperal fever epidemic at the Hotel Dieu in Paris during the 1780s, implies that they could, at times, be compliant:

> The midwife . . . to whose care the lying-in women are committed, was ordered to administer this remedy; and at whatever hour of the day or night the first symptoms of attack appeared she gave Ipecacuanha; and the success was in every instance the same; so that in four months during which this epidemic raged with fury, near two hundred women were saved to society, excepting five or six who all refused to take the vomit, and were victims of their own obstinacy.[24]

It is interesting to observe that, as nurses became more compliant, some patients might continue to be obstinate. It is difficult to see this excerpt from Whitehead's treatise as providing evidence for anything other than a taming of midwives and monthly nurses in the lying-in hospitals, which was mirrored half a century later by the taming of nurses in the Nightingale training schools and the London teaching hospitals.[25] Here are midwives following instructions – in France at any rate, if not in Britain. One adjunct to Whitehead's discussion of the use of hospital nurses to give prescribed remedies was his debate about whether nurses were intelligent enough to be trusted to administer medications.[26]

One variation from the almost entirely negative views expressed by physicians on the abilities of nurses can be found in Ferguson's 1839 treatise, *Essays on the Most Important Diseases of Women*. He observed:

> The late matron of the [general lying-in] hospital, Mrs Wright, remarked the effect of the hospital diet on the patients as often very depressing; and knowing, from the habits of this class of people, that gin was to many of them the common substitute for meat, she was induced to change the hospital dietary for a caudle in which gin was the staple. We shortly after this had a marked diminution in the intensity of the epidemic.[27]

Another reference to the same Mrs Wright can be found in the writings of Ferguson's older contemporary, Robert Gooch, who argued that one of the difficulties encountered when treating patients in lying-in hospitals was the reluctance of nurses to report ill-health to the physician. Gooch speculated that the heroic nature of the physicians' remedies might have something to do with this reticence:

The patients of a lying-in hospital are slow to confess themselves ill; they look upon pain of the belly as nothing but after-pains, and dread the active remedies which a confession of illness brings upon them; even after the confession the nurses are often dilatory in communicating it, and thus many hours used often to pass before I was called to the case, notwithstanding the activity, intelligence, and rare humanity of Mrs Wright, the matron.[28]

Such expressions of approval are rare in the medical writings. In fact, most physicians were extremely scathing[29] and their opinions could be summed up by the following extract from the work of John Clarke:

The care of persons in this state has been, till within the last century, almost exclusively confined to midwives, so that as a science midwifery may be considered to be still in its infancy – men of education having been rarely consulted, and then only in extraordinary cases of midwifery, it can hardly be a matter of surprise that so few observations connected with the practice of it are to be found in their works, and that improvement in this branch of medicine should not have kept pace with that of others.[30]

So the problem with traditional midwifery for the physicians of the eighteenth century was that it was not scientific, and that was because they – physicians – were not sufficiently engaged in its practice. They anticipated that now that 'men of learning' had control of this area of practice there would be a marked improvement in the general state of health of lying-in women.

THE RESPONSES OF THE MIDWIVES

What were the opinions of female midwives on these issues? Unfortunately, there is less written evidence giving their perspective. Although there are a great many works relating to this subject written by medical men between the years 1760 and 1850, there appear to have been few eighteenth-century treatises written by women to deal with similar issues. The most important of the writings by traditional midwives are Sarah Stone's *A Complete Practice of Midwifery* and Elizabeth Nihell's *A Treatise on the Art of Midwifery*.[31] Neither of these deals directly with puerperal fever, a subject that the female midwives undoubtedly saw as part of the physicians' area of expertise. Rather, they offer more general commentary on safe midwifery practice. Given the poor educational standard and the restricted publishing opportunities for women during this period it is not at all surprising that works by women were rare. Indeed, it seems extraordinary that any women published treatises on childbirth at this time.

One significant element of the treatises of Sarah Stone and Elizabeth Nihell is the forthright nature of their stated opinions of the work of the men-midwives; these statements can be interpreted as 'counter-attacks'. Sarah Stone, writing in 1737, commented on the tendency of men-midwives to rely on morbid anatomy rather than on experience and learned skills. She also gave voice to the resentment, no doubt felt by the majority of female midwives, at the tendency of men-midwives to claim credit at their expense. In her *Complete Practice of Midwifery* of 1737, she attempted to offer advice to female midwives about how to deal with difficult labours and deliveries, observing that there is no reason why they should not be able to handle a range of problems. She deplored the fact that they, too frequently, called in surgeons or men-midwives when they could have solved a problem themselves with a little more application and knowledge than they were using at present.[32] She added her scathing opinion of the men-midwives:

> Tis arrived to that height already, that almost every young Man who hath served his Apprenticeship to a Barber-Surgeon, immediately sets up for a Man-Midwife; altho' as ignorant, and, indeed, much ignoranter than the meanest woman of the Profession.[33]

Using terms that leave the reader in no doubt of her contempt for the male practitioners Stone further observed:

> These young Gentlemen Professors put on a finish'd assurance, with pretence that their knowledge exceeds any Woman's, because they have seen or gone thro' a Course of Anatomy: and so, if the Mother, or Child, or both die, as it often happens, they die Secundum Artem; for a Man was there, and the Woman-Midwife bears all the blame. Then it is that our young and well-assured pretenders boast, had they been there soon, neither should have died. Tho' I have made it my observation within these few years, That more women and Children have died by the hands of such Professors, than by the greatest imbecillity and ignorance of some Women-Midwives, who never went thro' or so much as heard of, a Course of Anatomy.[34]

Clearly, the message she wants to convey is that man-midwives are misleading both the public and themselves in their claims to superior knowledge based on an anatomical education. Here, it is possible to catch sight of an opposing view to that of the physicians, with their claims to knowledge that is both progressive and intrinsically 'enlightened' and 'scientific'. Stone continues:

> For give me leave to tell those young Gentlemen pretenders, who undertake the Practice of Midwifery with only the knowledge of dissecting the Dead, that all the Living who have or shall come under their care, in any difficulty, have and may severely pay for what knowledge they attain to in the Art of Midwifery . . . For dissecting the Dead, and being just and tender to the Living, are vastly different.[35]

The midwife Elizabeth Nihell, writing in 1760, refers to the medical treatise writers in similar terms to Sarah Stone, as 'so many authors who have, with the utmost confidence and the utmost absurdity, written upon the art of midwifery, without understanding anything at all of it.'[36] Like Stone she appears to want to convey the opinion that the knowledge claimed by the medical practitioners is spurious. She goes on to add that in claiming superior knowledge, the man-mid-wives are perpetrating a cynical confidence trick on society:

> But if they so falsely exalt their own learning above the ignorance of women; they have their reason for it. They seek to drive out of the practice those who stand in the way of their private interest: that private interest, to which the public one is forever sacrificed under the specious and stale pretext of its advancement.[37]

Again, alongside Sarah Stone, Nihell observes that female midwives are partly to blame for the male 'takeover' of midwifery practice. If they were willing to apply themselves to ensuring that their knowledge and skills were adequate, male practitioners would not be able to claim pre-eminence over them. The latter would, indeed, not even be able to get a 'foot in the door', if childbearing women were fully content with the female practitioners. She nevertheless believes that the claims of the man-midwives, along with their eagerness to intervene in deliveries, make them dangerous.[38]

CONCLUSION

Puerperal fever proved to be intractable for both traditional midwives and medical men during the eighteenth and early nineteenth centuries. It continued to pose an insurmountable problem until germ theory in the late nineteenth century, and the discovery of sulphonamides and penicillin in the first half of the twentieth, opened the way to a solution. During the period when medical theories abounded but no real answers could be found, two essentially very different groups of practitioners found themselves (although often working together in practice) to be frequently in a state of ideological and theoretical conflict. This was a conflict for which the often university-trained medical men were well equipped. Their social status and their superior education gave them an advantage over the humble traditional midwives. There were, however, among the latter, a small number who were able to challenge the men-midwives on their own terms. Sarah Stone and Elizabeth Nihell were successful in publishing treatises that, although not as eloquent or theoretically complex as the medical works, nevertheless offered a coherent and compelling defence of traditional practice.

And what of the patients? It is easy, with the benefit of hindsight, to observe that neither the bleeding and purging of the medical men nor the caudles of the traditional midwives are likely to have had any impact on puerperal fever. There is an irony for the modern reader in the recognition that it was not, finally, medical science but the serendipitous 'trial and error' work of biologists and chemists that finally opened the way to a cure. Perhaps in the final analysis, although they offer little insight into the disease itself, the eighteenth- and nineteenth-century writ-ings on puerperal fever can illuminate the preconceptions and ambitions of the medical men who wrote them. The writings of traditional midwives – few though they are – offer a useful counterbalance.

NOTES

1 See, for example, I. Loudon, 'Childbirth', in W.F. Bynum and R. Porter (eds), *Companion Encyclopedia of the History of Medicine,* London: Routledge, 1993, pp. 1050–71; J. Donnison, *Midwives and Medical Men: a History of the Struggle for the Control of Childbirth,* 2nd edn, London: Historical Publications Ltd, 1988; A. Wilson, *The Making of Man-midwifery: Childbirth in England, 1660–1770,* London: UCL Press, 1995, pp. 25–59; H. Roberts (ed.), *Women, Health and Reproduction,* London: Routledge and Kegan Paul, 1981; E. Shorter, *A History of Women's Bodies,* New York: Basic Books, 1982, Ch. 6.

2 Donnison, *Midwives and Medical Men;* Wilson, *The Making of Man-midwifery;* Loudon, 'Childbirth'.

3 G. Lawrence, 'Surgery (Traditional)', in Bynum, and Porter, 1993, *Companion Encyclopedia,* pp. 961–93. On apprenticeship, see J. Lane, 'The role of apprenticeship in eighteenth-century medical education in England', in W. F. Bynum and R. Porter (eds), *William Hunter and the Eighteenth-century Medical World,* Cambridge: Cambridge University Press, 1985, pp. 57–104.

4 T. Gelfand, 'The history of the medical profession', in Bynum and Porter, 1993, *Companion Encyclopedia,* pp. 1119–34.

5 On the education of men-midwives, see Bynum and Porter, 1985, *William Hunter,* pp. 343–69.

6 On eighteenth-century medicine and medical theory, see A. Cunningham, and R. French, *The Medical Enlightenment of the Eighteenth Century,* Cambridge: Cambridge University Press, 1990; and S. Lawrence, 'Medical education', in Bynum and Porter, 1993, *Companion Encyclopedia,* pp. 1151–79.

7 For a detailed discussion of these practices and their social implications, see: Wilson, *Making of Man-midwifery.* On traditional practices, see also: M. Bennett, 'Part one: Childbirth and infancy', in *Scottish Customs From the Cradle to the Grave,* Edinburgh: Polygon, 1992, pp. 1–77; and D. Buchan (ed.), *Folk Tradition and Folk Medicine in Scotland: the Writings of David Rorie,* Edinburgh: Canongate, 1994. On the issue of the autonomy of midwifery practice, see also: A. Friedman, 'Midwifery: legal or illegal? A case study of an accused, 1905', in C. Maggs (ed.), *Nursing History: the State of the Art.* London: Croom Helm, 1987, pp. 74–87.

8 Loudon, 'Childbirth'.

9 C. White, *A Treatise on the Management of Pregnant and Lying-in Women,* London: 1773, reprinted in F. Churchill (ed.), *Essays on the Puerperal Fever and Other Diseases Peculiar to Women, Selected from the Writings of British Authors Previous to the Close of the Eighteenth Century,* London: 1849, p. 231. The 'nurses' White refers to appear to be 'monthly nurses', who cared for women after delivery, rather than midwives who delivered them. They were not midwives yet they appeared to provoke similar opposition.

10 Ibid., p. 231.

11 R. W. Johnson, *Friendly Cautions to the Heads of Families and Others,* the first American edition. Philadelphia, 1804; Anonymous, *The Domestic Pharmacopoeia.* London: 1805; T. Ewell, *The Ladies' Medical Companion,* Philadelphia, 1818; Anonymous, *The Accomplished Ladies' Rich Closet of Rarities,* 3rd edn, London: 1691; Anonymous ('By a physician') *The Ladies' Physical Directory,* London: 1739; J. Maubray, *The Female Physician,* London: 1724.

12 G. Armstrong, *An Account of the Diseases Most Incident to Children . . . To Which is Added an Essay on Nursing,* London: 1777; Anonymous, *The Art of Nursing: or the Method of Bringing up Young Children,* 2nd edn, London: 1733; J. Astruc, (transl.) *A General and Compleat Treatise on all the Diseases Incident to Children,* London: 1746; W. Cadogan, *An Essay upon Nursing,* London: 1772; W. Moss, A*n Essay on the Management and Nursing of Children,* London: 1781; Anonymous, *Observations*

Upon the Proper Nursing of Children, London: 1761; J. Kennedy, *Instructions to Mothers and Nurses*, Glasgow, 1825; H. Jenner, *A Guide to Mothers and Nurses*, London: 1826; W. Rowley, *Dr Rowley's Treatise*, London: 1801; H. Smith, *Letters to Married Women on Nursing and the Management of Children*, London: 1792; H. W. Tytler, *Paedotrophia; or the Art of Nursing*, London: 1797; C. F. Vandenburgh, *The Mother's Medical Guardian*, London: 1820. Please note that there is also an interesting example of a treatise on nursing written by a nurse, Mrs Hanbury: *The Good Nurse*, London: Longman, 1825.

13   T. Dawkes, *The Midwife Rightly Instructed*, London: 1736; J. Astruc (transl.) *The Art of Midwifery Reduced to Principles*, London: 1767. In his treatise, Astruc offers advice to the physician on how to make midwifery works simple enough for midwives to understand, pp. 6–7; *Aristotle's Compleat and Experienced Midwife* (transl. William Salmon), London: 1749; Anonymous, *Sanctioned by her Majesty's Example . . . The British Ladies Institution*, London: 1806. A text by Nicholas Culpeper, first published in 1651 also went through numerous corrections and reprints during the second half of the eighteenth century: N. Culpeper, *A Directory for Midwives*, London: 1651; Anonymous, *A Directory for Midwives . . . Newly Corrected*, London: 1755; Anonymous, *A Directory for Midwives*, London: 1777.

14   T. Reid, *An Essay on the Nature and Cure of the Phthisis Pulmonalis*, London: 1782, pp. 15–17. On this issue, as it relates to lying-in women, see P. P. Walsh, *Practical Observations on the Puerperal Fever*, London: 1787, p. 55. Debate in the literature regarding the quality of work of midwives and nurses can be found in: D. N. Harley, 'Ignorant Midwives – a persistent stereotype', *Society for the Social History of Medicine Bulletin*, 1980, Vol. 26, pp. 6–9; S. A. Seligman, 'The Royal maternity charity: the first hundred years', *Medical History*, 1980, Vol. 24, pp. 403–18; H. Marland (ed.), *The Art of Midwifery: Early Modern Midwives in Europe*, London: Routledge, 1993; H. Marland and A. M. Rafferty (eds), *Midwives, Society and Childbirth: Debates and Controversies in the Early Modern Period*, London: Routledge, 1997; M. J. Van Lieburg, G. J. Kloosterman, *'Mother and Child were Saved': the Memoirs (1693–1740) of the Frisian Midwife Catharina Schrader*, Amsterdam: Rodopi, 1987.

15   J. Clarke, *Practical Essays on the Management of Pregnancy and Labour*, London: 1793.

16   J. Sharp, *The Midwives' Book*, London: 1671; S. Stone, *Complete Practice of Midwifery*, London: 1737; E. Nihell, *Treatise on the Art of Midwifery*, London: 1760. For comment on Sharp's work, see I. Grundy, 'Sarah Stone: enlightenment midwife', in R. Porter, *Medicine in the Enlightenment*, Amsterdam: Rodopi, 1995, pp. 128–144. For an example of a woman writing an apparently very popular general health manual see M. Johnson, *Madam Johnson's Present*, London: 1755. For an example of an early modern French midwife who wrote on obstetrical issues, see W. Perkins, *Midwifery and Medicine in Early Modern France: Louise Bourgeois*, Exeter: Exeter University Press, 1996. Bourgeios wrote, among other works, *Observations diverses sur la sterilite-perte de fruict foecondite accouchements et maladies des femmes et enfants nouveaux naiz*, Paris: 1626. This work focuses on some medical issues of the day as well as on the 'art' of midwifery.

17   Jane Sharp referred to childbed fever: Sharp, *The Midwives' Book*, Ch. III, 'Of Feavers after Child-bearing', pp. 243–5.

18   C. White, *An Appendix to the Second Edition of Mr. White's Treatise on the Management of Pregnant and Lying-in Women*, London: 1777, in Churchill, *Essays on the puerperal fever*, pp. 268–71.

19   Ibid., p. 270.

20   Ibid., p. 271. White cites numerous other similar cases. See, in particular, Case VI, pp. 276–7.

21   A. Gordon, *A Treatise on the Epidemic Puerperal Fever of Aberdeen*, London: 1795, p. 6.

22 Ibid., p. 30.

23 J. Armstrong, *Facts and Observations Relative to the Fever Commonly called Puerperal,* London: 1814, pp. 42–3.

24 J. Whitehead, *A Report Made by Order of the Government,* London: 1783, p. 10.

25 My assertion that nurses were 'tamed' in the nineteenth century is, of course, highly interpretative. On the history of nursing more generally, see A. M. Rafferty, *The Politics of Nursing Knowledge,* London: Routledge, 1996; C. Maggs, 'A general history of nursing: 1800–1900', in Bynum and Porter, 1993, *Companion Encyclopedia,* pp. 1309–28. R. Dingwall, A. M. Rafferty and C. Webster, *An Introduction to the Social History of Nursing,* London: Routledge, 1988; G. Hardy, *William Rathbone and the Early History of District Nursing,* Ormskirk: G. W. & A. Hesketh, 1981; A. H. Jones (ed.), *Images of Nurses,* Philadelphia: University of Pennsylvania Press, 1988; S. D. Krampitz, 'Nursing power, nursing politics', in Maggs, *State of the Art,* pp. 60–73; C. Maggs, *The Origins of General Nursing,* London: Croom Helm, 1983; S. McGann, *The Battle of the Nurses,* London: Scutari, 1992; B. Mortimer, 'Independent women: domiciliary nurses in mid-nineteenth-century Edinburgh', in A. M. Rafferty, J. Robinson, and R. Elkan, *Nursing History and the Politics of Welfare,* London: Routledge, 1997, pp. 133–49. See also S. Hunt, and A. Symonds, *The Social Meaning of Midwifery,* Basingstoke: Macmillan, 1995.

26 Whitehead, Report of the Government, p. viii.

27 R. Ferguson, *Essays on the Most Important Diseases of Women,* London: 1839, p. 168.

28 R. Gooch, *An Account of Some of the Most Important Diseases Peculiar to Women,* London: 1829. pp. 44–5.

29 See, for example, W. Campbell, *A Treatise on the Epidemic Puerperal fever,* Edinburgh, 1822, p. 4.

30 J. Clarke, *An Essay on the Epidemic Disease of Lying-in Women,* London: 1788, Preface. p. ii.

31 Stone, *Complete Practice of Midwifery*; Nihell, *Treatise on the Art of Midwifery*; one seventeenth-century treatise is also of interest in this context: Sharp *The midwives book*; see Wilson, *The Making of Man-midwifery* on Sarah Stone, pp. 57–59; and on Elizabeth Nihell, pp. 197–9.

32 Stone, *Complete Practice of Midwifery,* p. x.

33 Ibid., p. xi.

34 Ibid., pp. xi–xii

35 Ibid., p. xii.

36 Nihell, *Treatise on the Art of Midwifery,* p. ii

37 Ibid., p. vi

38 Ibid., p. viii–ix.

5 *Sanba* and their clients

Midwives and the medicalization of childbirth in Japan 1868 to *c*. 1920

Aya Homei

In 1868, after years of domestic political turmoil in Japan, the Meiji period (1868–1912) began and Japan launched itself as a modern nation state. The modern nation geared itself to mobilize people for modernization, a term that implied enlightenment and industrialization.[1]

As part of this scheme, the Meiji government also set out to modernize medical practitioners, a group they perceived as essential for national prosperity. In 1868, the government officially declared that Japanese medicine was to be modelled on modern Western, and especially German, medicine. Obstetric experts, including midwives, were part of this modernization programme and an early government directive of 1868 banned midwives from practising abortion and trading in drugs. In 1874, the officials implemented a Medical System (*isei*) in three major cities, which included three regulations that applied to midwives. These are thought to be the first regulations for midwives in Japan that defined midwives as modern medical professionals. From then on, local authorities developed their own midwifery regulations, which were later consolidated in the national Midwives Ordinance promulgated in 1899; this Ordinance made midwifery training, examination and local registration obligatory for all future midwives.

Under these conditions new obstetricians and midwives emerged slowly during the Meiji period. In the first half of the period, up to *c*. 1890, elite medical students interested in obstetrics travelled to Germany to study Prussian obstetrics and gynaecology. On their return to Japan, from the late 1880s onwards, they taught German scientific midwifery to female students. Graduates of these formal midwifery training schools were commonly known as *shin-sanba* ('new-midwives') or *seiyô-sanba* ('Western midwives') to distinguish them from indigenous *kyû-sanba* ('old-midwives') or the old-style *toriagebaba*, who conducted midwifery based on skills they had acquired through experience, not medical training.

Toriagebaba, or the 'old woman who pulls and lifts the baby', were survivals of pre-modern Japan. In this earlier period, the Edo period (1603–1867), a Japanese version of scientific obstetrics was in place, and obstetricians were primarily involved in the management of difficult childbirth and births among noble or court families. Among the remaining population, *toriagebaba* attended almost all non-problematic childbirths. These attendants were usually senior members of the community, experienced in childbirth and the traditional duties of birth attendants. The British equivalent of Japanese *toriagebaba* were the so-called handywomen or granny midwives.[2] When labour began, the family invited a *toriagebaba* to the private birth room or the community birth hut, where female relatives (in some regions close male kin were included) and neighbours assisted the birthing woman and *toriagebaba*. Some of these attendants lived entirely on the proceeds of their midwifery practice, whereas for others this was an occasional occupation.[3]

The altered political environment of the Meiji period and the emergence of modern medical birth attendants introduced change into the established local birthing cultures. The medical *shin-sanba* typically required the parturient woman to adopt the supine birth position, used chemical disinfectants to wash her hands and the birthing woman's genitalia and carried a professional-looking leather bag that contained the 'midwife's seven tools', which included a catheter, gauze and ligatures. Finally, the *shin-sanba* justified their new practices as modern medicine.

Besides these new obstetric practices, their role in the newly emerged nation state differentiated *shin-sanba* from their predecessors, the *toriagebaba*. Early Meiji officials were desperate to introduce and incorporate modern hygiene into Japanese lives. They hoped that midwives would popularize the concept by disseminating it to birthing women. Another responsibility of the *shin-sanba* emerged in the second decade of the twentieth century. By this time Japan had experienced modern warfare and the government expected *shin-sanba* to assist in improving the 'national physique' by securing the birth of healthy children.[4]

Following the efforts of the government and supporters of the *shin-sanba*, the number of *shin-sanba* grew and, by around 1910, they exceeded the number of *kyû-sanba*. Subsequent events further advantaged the professionalization of *shin-sanba* and, by the end of the Second World War, educated medical *sanba* became the norm even in many remote areas.

Behind this apparently smooth and comparatively swift modernization of midwives, regional birth culture itself changed slowly. People preserved idiosyncratic, pre-modern local rituals, they continued to practise abortion and infanticide, albeit illegally, and – worst of all for *shin-sanba* – they continued to hire *kyû-sanba*.[5] The bitter reality faced by the modern birth attendants is revealed in the pages of *Josan no Shiori*, the first and longest surviving monthly professional midwifery journal in modern Japan that was founded by Ogata Masakiyo, a Prussian-trained obstetrician–gynaecologist.

OGATA MASAKIYO AND *JOSAN NO SHIORI*

Ogata Masakiyo

Ogata Masakiyo (1864–1919) was born in Kagawa Prefecture in 1864, during the political turmoil that preceded the Meiji period. In 1879 he entered the Takamatsu Medical School. Two years later, he moved to Tokyo and entered the Special Course of the Medical Department at the University of Tokyo. While still a student he married a granddaughter of Ogata Kôan, renowned physician and founder of a leading school in Osaka. At this time he adopted his wife's family name of

Ogata. In 1887, having completed his medical studies, he began to work at the Private Ogata Hospital in Osaka. In 1888, Ogata went to Germany to study obstetrics under such eminent university obstetricians as Professor Bernhard Sigismund Schultze of Jena; he was awarded a degree in Freiburg with a thesis on the history of Japanese midwifery. Ogata returned to Osaka in March 1892 after three years in Europe, and was promoted to head of the department of obstetrics and gynaecology at Ogata Hospital. At around the same time, he was appointed principal at the Medical School at Osaka Jikei Hospital. In 1902 Ogata founded his own clinic, Ogata Women's Hospital.

Ogata was a powerful figure locally and nationally, within and beyond the community of obstetricians. In local politics he once served on the Osaka City Assembly; in the medical world, he was a founder member of the Kansai Society for Obstetrics and Gynaecology, which was launched in April 1899, and of the half-public, half-private Osaka branch of the Greater Japan Private Hygiene Society;[6] and he was also president of the Osaka Medical Association. At national level, he was one of seventeen delegates appointed by the government to observe the International Congress of Medicine in Portugal in 1909.[7] Ogata also led the champions of *shin-sanba* in his region. Inspired by the German system, he opened the Ogata Midwifery School in June 1892, three months after his return from Germany. Following the establishment of the Osaka Midwives' Association in 1899, he served as the first President.[8] Finally, he campaigned to modify the name of trained *sanba* to the neutral *josanpu* ('female birth attendant'), rather than *sanba* ('old woman of birth'), which Ogata considered to be pre-modern.[9]

'On the Reform of Midwives'

In 1896, Ogata launched a professional seminar/lecture group at Ogata Hospital, The Midwifery Society. He hoped that in this forum *josanpu* would exchange ideas on modern practices of medical midwifery with colleagues and their obstetric teachers. Only fifty-three people participated in the first meeting in May 1896, but a year later the numbers attending had risen tenfold. In 1900, one year after the promulgation of the Midwives' Ordinance, the number of participants was 700. In January 1897, the Society nominated six prominent obstetrician–gynaecologists, including Hamada Gentatsu, the leading practitioner in Meiji Japan, to be honorary members. Later, in October 1910, thirty prominent foreign obstetrician–gynaecologists were made honorary members.[10]

Ogata was aware that poor transportation made it impossible for a number of his graduates who lived in distant parts of Japan to attend the Society conferences. For those suburban and provincial *josanpu*, Ogata and his colleagues published the Society's monthly professional journal, *Josan no Shiori* (*Guide to Midwifery*). This journal, launched in June 1896, was published continuously until 1944. The first issue was circulated to 200 subscribers, who automatically became Society members; in 1913, the journal had 1,118 subscribers, and by 1916, over 2,000 copies were distributed. Government agents received complimentary copies, a copy of the first issue was sent to the Central Hygiene Bureau, and after August 1897, a copy went to each prefecture's Hygiene Department.

In the opening article of the first issue of *Josan no Shiori*, Ogata wrote 'On the Reform of Midwives'.[11] Although the title referred only to the reform of midwives, throughout the text Ogata demanded the reform or modernization of others involved in obstetric care. In this group he included old-style obstetricians, health policy makers and lay people. During the 1890s, elite obstetricians were working to transform their discipline by adopting the principles and practices of German medicine and detaching themselves from pre-modern Edo. Yet Ogata believed this action to be insufficient, and proposed that obstetrician–gynaecologists who truly wished their discipline to be recognized as modern needed to influence others whose ideas and actions shaped their professional domain.

THE MODERN AS A MODEL: CASE HISTORIES FROM NEW-MIDWIVES

Josan no Shiori was a vehicle that broadcast Ogata's modern messages, it became an important medium through which the modernization of Japanese midwifery was promoted. With this end in view, editors in the early years translated and published modern German case histories that emphasized the value of disinfection and the select referral of abnormal clients to physicians for further treatment. These German cases were presented as models, with the specific intention of guiding the reader in a certain direction. *Josan no Shiori* expected Japan's new midwives to be vigilant in the supervision of normal birth, to practise meticulous hygiene, and to entrust abnormal cases to obstetrician–gynaecologists.[12]

In time midwives, both urban and rural, began to submit their case histories to the section called *jikken*, the 'case study'.[13] This soon became a significant part of the journal and was allocated many pages by the editors. The section was illustrated with a picture of a baby holding a banner that said '*jikken* is our teacher'. The merits of the section were clear; *jikken* was designed to supplement the inexperience of 'new midwives'. Through *jikken*, city and rural midwives became familiar with the variety of cases each experienced; this sort of professional exchange was not possible for the traditional, local *toriagebaba*.

The Japanese case histories copied the writing style of the German case histories; the German style was also characteristic of the rest of the journal. For instance, *josanpu* and regular reporter, Morita Makiko (from Hiroshima), gave an account of her experience with a breech presentation in the October 1910 issue.[14] According to Morita, a nineteen-year-old woman in her seventh month of pregnancy visited her for the first time on 26 June. Morita examined her and realized that the uterine fundus was very high. She suspected a transverse presentation and 'suggested that she should get a doctor's check-up'.[15] A doctor came, attempted to turn the fetus and claimed to have corrected the infant's position. Later, on 19 July, Morita was called to the labour. Morita arrived several hours later and, after external and stethoscope examinations, with 'disinfected hands and fingers made an internal examination'.[16] Morita then found that the cervix was fully dilated and that a limb was already descending. However, she 'did not manage to discern whether it was a lower or upper extremity,' so she 'asked family members to call on an obstetrician'.[17] At nine o'clock, three hours after Morita's arrival at the house, the infant's legs appeared at the vulva, just when the obstetrician finally arrived. The obstetrician then successfully delivered the infant. The delivery was completed at 9.25 p.m. but the infant was in a critical condition. Morita used a catheter to remove mucus from the baby's airways and began resuscitation, which eventually saved the baby.

Morita's case followed the German model accounts and demonstrated the dichotomized division of labour among modern medical practitioners. Modern, medical *sanba* practised the care and supervision of normal birth but as soon as complications occurred, obstetricians were called in to resolve abnormal cases by manipulation. The story can be interpreted as a success story of modern medicine. Accounts in this genre depicted medical treatment saving both mother and infant, they also contributed to the construction of an image of reliable *shin-sanba*.

CONSTRUCTION OF THE DANGEROUS AND IGNORANT PRE-MODERN

In the decades that began in 1890, obstetrician–gynaecologists started to work on producing new midwives. In 1910, the ratio of new- to old- midwives was inverted, and new midwives began to submit case histories of childbirth problems attributed to the actions of *kyû-sanba*. In the sixth issue of *Josan no Shiori*, in November 1896, a new-midwife from Miyazaki and a graduate of Ogata Midwifery Training School, Matsuyama Tomiko, recounted a case of puerperal infection.[18] A doctor had asked her to visit a woman during her lying-in period. Matsuyama found a twenty-two-year-old woman with 'pale complexion, exhausted and sometimes in extreme pain'.[19] According to the family, a *kyû-sanba* had attended the woman's delivery. The birth went very smoothly but afterwards the woman felt pulsating pain in her vulva, which stung intensely during urination. Three days after the labour, the vulva was swollen and the pain had become too extreme to sleep peacefully. The family consulted with the *kyû-sanba* but she 'did not take it particularly seriously so she did not make any examination'.[20] Seven days later, the family talked to a doctor specializing in indigenous medicine. He also claimed that the problem was quite common, spread oil on the mother's vulva and left. Her condition deteriorated further and Matsuyama was finally asked to examine her. She checked the vagina and diagnosed 'second stage [vaginal] rupture'. She also 'saw a grand tumour around the vagina and on the injured surface a very rotten-smelling secretion had accumulated'.[21] Having seen the condition, Matsuyama 'cleansed the injured part carefully as well as inside of the vagina with 100 times diluted lukewarm Lysol solution, spread iodoform, attached gauze soaked in boric acid, bandaged the part with a T-bandage, and returned home'.[22] Thereafter, Matsuyama cared for the woman every day and, as a result of her efforts, two weeks later the woman was able to walk around her garden.

The *josanpu* writing for the journal also criticized clients, usually the closest kin of the birthing women, including the male head of the family, who held authority over the selection of birth attendants.[23] Morita again published an account, in the September 1899 issue, of a case in which a 'healthy farmer from Minami-Village, Hiroshima, who had previously delivered four times' passed away following a delivery first attended by an aged midwife.[24] On 26 July 1899 the woman experienced labour pains but the infant did not appear; the client family called on Morita. She described: 'haemorrhage had left her white faced, with a weak pulse, and acutely anaemic, despite these conditions, the old non-licensed midwife forced the woman to assume a squatting position. This treatment was standard practice for an old-midwife but in this instance it caused more bleeding, cerebral anaemia, and vomiting'.[25] Morita lay the woman flat, lowered her head and ordered her to rest. Having detected no sign of life in the abdomen by external examination and with stethoscope, Morita then 'disinfected fingers and hands' and performed an internal examination. As a result, she recognized placenta praevia. As a first-aid measure, Morita pressed a tampon into the vagina while pleading to the family to call an obstetrician. The doctor came, confirmed Morita's diagnosis and performed internal version; unfortunately the baby was stillborn. The mother remained frail; the doctor prescribed her a stimulant but she passed away on the following day. After the story, Morita commented:

> We already know about the danger of placenta praevia from our dear teachers. In a remote area, it is common that one rarely sees good midwives; therefore people trust ignorant non-licensed or old midwives who do not know anything about the horror of haemorrhage. They assume that much bleeding means that the labour is progressing, and family members usually do not dream of the dangerous consequence of it. Only when I examined the woman did [the woman's family] get to know the danger. The presence of the doctor was ultimately unsuccessful. I truly cannot bear to see a family experience the tragedy of losing both mother and infant.[26]

Although Morita acknowledged the situation in remote areas that compelled lay people to employ 'ignorant' 'old-midwives' and expressed sympathy for the distressing consequences, she also subtly belittled the family because people in her area 'usually do not dream of the dangerous consequence of hiring old-midwives' and that this particular client family called Morita, a good midwife, too late. In this sense, old-midwives and these clients were equally criticized for their ignorance about modern childbirth and midwifery. To Morita, anything pre-modern – or even non-modern – was scorned.

This ongoing stigmatization of the 'pre-modern' by modern new-midwives during this period went hand in hand with the elite obstetrician–gynaecologists' claim that midwives owed a duty to the nation. *Josan no Shiori* printed the speech that a physician Yoshida Kentarô, from Fukuoka, gave at Ogata's alumni union in 1899. He recounted an anecdote in which a *kyû-sanba* misjudged the situation and allowed a woman to develop a critical condition. He said: 'this kind of incompetent midwife is truly a social-moral criminal who prevents the foundation of a "rich nation with strong soldiers" (*fukoku kyôhei*)', thus hinting that the professionalism of new-midwives was a prediction of the success of the nation.[27] In the 1909 issue of *Josan no Shiori*, Takahashi Shingorô, Ogata's first disciple and a vigorous supporter of the new-midwife in the remote northern Niigata prefecture, argued the case for the provision of subsidies to new-midwives in rural areas, he made use of vital statistics:

> The infant mortality rate in our country is the highest [compared to Western countries] and if we compare this to the hygienically most advanced country, Germany, it is triple the number. The incompetence of midwives results in the unnecessary death many infants. This results in the loss to Japan of 94,700 infant lives every year; this loss can only be remedied by the development and modernization of midwives.[28]

By the beginning of the twentieth century Japan had experienced two major wars, the Sino-Japanese War (1894–5) and the Russo-Japanese War (1904–5). These experiences had made the government acutely aware of the health of its citizens. Specifically, when officials prepared for the 1911 International Hygiene Exposition in Dresden, they recognized Japan's high maternal mortality rates as compared to Western countries.[29] As a result, in 1916, the government launched *hoken eisei chôsakai*, the 'committee for the investigation of people's health and hygiene', and hired local officials and physicians to scrutinize the comparative quality of the Japanese *Kokutai*, 'national physique'. In this context, prominent obstetrician–gynaecologists, like Takahashi, used the population rhetoric to promote modern scientific midwifery, as they claimed this strategy would meet the national need.

THE REALITY IN THE FIELD

Kyû-sanba and *shin-sanba*

In spite of the hostility expressed by *shin-sanba/josanpu* towards *kyû-sanba* in the published case histories, the narratives also reveal that *kyû-sanba* and *shin-sanba* were often both present in the Meiji birth scene. Lay clients generally continued to hire *kyû-sanba* for the overall supervision of the childbirth process, and those who could afford modern medical care called on *shin-sanba* when critical complications occurred.

This dual structure was partly enforced by the realities of the modern medical system in Japan. Throughout the modern period, the government regulated medicine and modelled this regulation on German practice, but the government did not interfere with the *laissez faire* nature of the medical market.[30] Consequently, educated obstetrician–gynaecologists chose to practise in urban areas inhabited by the well-to-do.[31] They opened clinics for wealthy or middle-class families willing to pay for modern medical treatment. As a result, few doctors were available for the majority of the Japanese population living in the rural areas. In this situation, *shin-sanba* were the possessors of modern medical knowledge and skills in the remote areas, where they took the place of the doctors.

The early generations of *shin-sanba* had not only invested their capital in training, they had also purchased medical instruments and other expensive equipment, such as bicycles and telephones, to make their work easier.[32] The end result was that they charged more than the *kyû-sanba* for their services. Another feature of these *shin-sanba* could be problematic for potential clients of lower social standing: the early *shin-sanba* were normally members of middle-class ex-samurai families, and this alone might cause more humble clients to reject their services. *Kyû-sanba*, on the other hand, were inexpensive, accessible to a wider population and flexible with regard to payment. In addition, most of the *kyû-sanba* were from the same community as their clients and had already established a relationship with members of the community. Clients also respected the *kyû-sanba*'s experience, while discrediting the relative youth and practical inexperience of *shin-sanba*.[33] These factors were sufficiently powerful to result in the development of a two-tiered system of birth attendance during the Meiji period.

Unusual allies

Paradoxically, that section of the journal in which *josanpu* vigorously constructed the binary image of 'safe, virtuous, modern medical new-midwives' in contrast to 'dangerous, vicious, pre-modern old-midwives', also warmly accommodated the *kyû-sanba* who attempted to modernize themselves. A letter to Ogata from a country 'new-midwife', Kobayashi Hisa, told that in her village, some *kyû-sanba* were being 'renewed'. Kobayashi acquainted herself with a *kyû-sanba*, one of the 'most modernized among the old ones,' who called on her whenever she judged the pregnancy to be abnormal.[34] In her letter, Kobayashi explained the virtue of modernized *kyû-sanba* by emphasizing the danger of other *kyû-sanba* who jeopardized the birthing woman because they stuck to pre-modern customs. Integral to her attitude was the assumption that modern was good. The modern was so virtuous and powerful that it had the power to nullify whatever dangerous elements the *kyû-sanba* had formerly embodied.

Kobayashi's letter also pointed to the diversity among *kyû-sanba*, suggesting that the simple dichotomy of *shin-sanba* and *kyû-sanba* was in many cases invalid. In the early Meiji period, Japan nationally embraced, hailed and encouraged modernity for her citizens.[35] In the sphere of childbirth, during the early Meiji period when the number of modern medical birth practitioners was insufficient to diffuse the concept of modern hygienic childbirth, local health officers attempted to modernize *toriagebaba* by intensive courses in midwifery theory. As a result, a number of *kyû-sanba* became *shin-sanba* by passing the midwifery examination.[36] They were familiar with modern medicine and able to communicate with the medically trained yet practically inexperienced *shin-sanba* who appeared in later years. *Shin-sanba* appreciated such modernized *kyû-sanba*; they could be valuable allies, able to introduce *shin-sanba* to clients.

Such alliances between *kyû-sanba* and *shin-sanba* became common in later years and some *shin-sanba* appropriated local knowledge from *kyû-sanba*. Mrs C, born in 1918, remembered that she learned practical wisdom from a *toriagebaba* in her village in Kumano.[37] Mrs C first studied nursing at Ogata's school in Osaka and acquired a midwifery licence in the late 1930s. She opened her business in 1946, when *toriagebaba* were still active primary birth attendants in her region. Mrs C was critical of the *toriagebaba* because they did not disinfect, yet she appropriated a *toriagebaba*'s experience-based suggestions: Mrs C asked one *toriagebaba*, 'some seventy-year-old who loved to chat', to instruct her in the *ko-shiyu* (literally, 'bathing up till the lower-back') technique. This technique aimed to accelerate labour. The birthing woman immersed herself in a tub full of hot water up to the stomach and the mother and tub were then covered by a cloth. The *koshiyu* would then warm and relax the birthing woman's body, making the delivery of the baby easier. It was quite a contrast to what Mrs C learned at the midwifery training school but, instead of dogmatically following the modern medical method, Mrs C decided to incorporate *koshiyu* technique in her practice.[38]

The reasons why *shin-sanba* befriended *toriagebaba* and adopted their 'wise' knowledge varied. Most plausibly, this occurred because the traditional knowledge would directly improve the *shin-sanba*'s business. In practice, whether the business would prosper or not was heavily dependent on whether a *shin-sanba* had sufficiently flexible skills and could adjust both to the demands of clients and to the local birth culture. The easiest way for *shin-sanba* to get to know the unique local conditions was by working directly with *kyû-sanba*. Developing good relationships with *kyû-sanba* would also bring other benefits to *shin-sanba*. *Kyû-sanba* might recommend *shin-sanba* to local women clients, and directly refer those clients to *shin-sanba* in cases of complications. *Toriagebaba* also profited from such collaboration. Although in the short term *toriagebaba* would not benefit economically as much as if they practised by themselves, in the long term they gained socially. In the delivery room, more than one medical practitioner customarily attended complicated deliveries in order to spread the grave responsibility.[39] Thus, by maintaining good terms with other birth practitioners, *toriagebaba* won their professional security at the cost of some of their income.

Less popular medical practitioners

The pattern of birth attendance was most problematic for modern male physicians. They were middle-class and expensive so many client households called on modern physicians or obstetric experts only as a last resort. A *shin-sanba* from Osaka, Ikegami Yoneko, wrote of a case where the client family persistently refused the obstetrician's treatment because of their poverty.[40] Against Ikegami's advice, the family persisted in postponing consultation with a doctor saying, 'in case of emergency, we will be rescued by a benevolent doctor so let us see the condition a little bit longer'.[41] Thus, in the end, Ikegami, although anxious about the progress of the delivery, gave in. Fortunately, three hours later, a live baby was born and the placenta followed twenty minutes later.

Although a common reason for the client's rejection of further medical treatment was expense, there were many other reasons. Ueda Teru, another 'new-midwife' from Osaka, described in the April 1905 issue a case of anencephaly and cleft palate in a twenty-one-year-old woman's infant.[42] The client family called Ueda for the first time in July, during the fifth month of pregnancy. The family followed the religion of Tenrikyô and had previously asked the Tenrikyô teacher for a diagnosis and further instructions.[43] But when the labour started in February 1905, the family called on Ueda, who examined the birthing woman, diagnosed an abnormal presentation and suggested consulting a physician. The family would not agree, so she was forced to do her best within the limits of her professional expertise.

Another reason for rejecting obstetricians was shame. Often, in the case of illegitimate pregnancy a woman's position attracted gossip, this was especially so in the countryside. Therefore, when an unmarried woman became pregnant her family usually preferred to avoid birth attendants or possible 'rumour spreaders'. New-midwife Takagaki Koto told of a case of triplets.[44] A twenty-three-year-old woman from Ikeda (a suburb of Osaka City) moved to Osaka for the first time in 1895, as a maid to a merchant family. She became pregnant, was dismissed by her employer and sent back to Ikeda. However, her family feared the gossip that her condition might provoke and she returned to Osaka to stay with a widow whom she knew.[45] Soon she suffered from a nutritional disorder, but even at this stage she 'neither pleaded for the doctor's treatment nor requested a [new] midwife's protection because she was depressed'.[46] When labour started, someone called Takagaki, who realized that a second opinion by an expert was absolutely essential. However, the family twice rejected the suggestion and the woman died.

As these case histories illustrate, modern obstetrician–gynaecologists or clinical physicians in general were in a difficult situation. Although their allies, the *shin-sanba*, tried hard to persuade clients to consult obstetricians, their suggestion was often rejected and the *shin-sanba* had to undertake difficult cases. The rejection of medical men stemmed partly from the *laissez faire* medical market but also from the view that modern physicians played a role as official vigilante in the community. This was particularly noticeable from the beginning of the twentieth century: state officials and middle-class citizens, each holding particular interests, allied together to 'socially manage' the Japanese population.[47] Religious groups that differed from the Shinto principle were condemned as pseudo religions or evil cults. The feminist movement from 1910 onwards demanded the recognition of common-law marriages but their efforts were marginalized, swamped by other forces that promoted the image of legally married women as the norm.[48] In this social milieu, it appears that some client families regarded the conformist obstetrician–gynaecologists as spies and thus avoided dealing with them. These client fears were in part justified because the government expected modern birth attendants, not only obstetrician–gynaecologists but also *shin-sanba,* to monitor all reproductive matters, especially abortion and infanticide, both of which became nationally illegal under the Meiji government.

Illicit reality: abortion and infanticide

In the Edo period, abortion and infanticide were as accepted a part of reproductive activities as pregnancy and childbirth.[49] Around the mid-Edo period, in response to widespread belief that abortion and infanticide would hinder economic development, some fiefs issued a ban on these practices. The fiefs of Sendai and Tsuyama were known to be most adamant, elaborating procedures that required people both to report pregnancies and births and to observe their neighbours' reproductive practices.[50] For the majority of the population, the illicit practices of abortion and infanticide continued to be regarded as essential responses to recurrent economic crises during the rest of the Edo period. However, the traditional practice clashed with a new view of the nature of life, which emerged in the eighteenth century. According to this new argument, after the fifth month of pregnancy the fetus was regarded as human. Thus, the population of the Edo period compromised over abortion in response to a range of circumstances, including economic pressure, the definition of life and the impact of official surveillance.[51]

In the Meiji period, along with the emergence of a modern legal system, infanticide and abortion were criminalized through *Shinritsu Kôryô* (The Essential of the New Law) and *Kaitei Ritsurei* (Amended Statutes and Sub-statutes) promulgated in 1871 and 1873 respectively.[52] Later, in 1888, the Abortion Criminal Law provided for the independent policing of abortion.[53] These new regulations regarded those individuals who had abortions, or who encouraged the practice, sold abortifacients or induced abortions, as criminally culpable.

Despite the legislation, people continued to have abortions and practise infanticide, as the following examples show. In the local court in Muraoka between 1879 and 1880, a case was heard on the allegation that Terakura Banzô's wife, Tatsu, had smothered their infant.[54] In 1880 and 1881, a fifty-one-year-old woman was found guilty and sentenced to three years' penal servitude for her involvement in the death of an infant born to Nishigaki Maki and his wife's niece.

Josan no Shiori confirmed the existence of such practices even after the 1890s. Under the title 'Abortion by An Old Woman Ogre', the journal reported that forty-two-year-old Chise, the wife of thirty-four-year-old Fukunaga Seikichi from Shika-Village, Banshû, was found to have aborted an infant in June 1911 with the assistance of an 'old house watcher' in the same village.[55] At the local court in Himeji, Chise confessed that she had intercourse with thirty-five-year-old Yamada Komimatsu from neighbouring Yongô-Village and became pregnant while her husband was away working in Korea. Chise consulted with the 'old house watcher', who was sympathetic to her and offered to perform an abortion.

As in Chise's case, clients asked local midwives to carry out the procedure. These midwives were often the *mumenkyo-sanba*, the 'non-licensed midwives' who were considered to belong to the *kyû-sanba*.[56] In November 1911, the journal published a brief account of a criminal abortion case in Chiba.[57] The large number of reports of stillborn and smothered babies led officers at the Regional Kinoshita Police Office to suspect illegal reproductive practices in their area. The officers singled out a report submitted on 21 October 1911 by Mrs Iwai Tatsu about her stillborn son. Shortly after, a police officer and a doctor, Mr Okuma, visited the Iwai family in Hongô-Village to interrogate the family. During the interview, Tatsu confessed that she had undergone an abortion assisted by a fifty-five-year-old *mumenkyo-sanba*, Yamasaki Oaki, from a neighbouring village. Yamasaki was arrested and admitted that she had learned the abortion technique thirty years before and that for the past two decades had practised it, without payment, in response to the demand from village women. She claimed to have induced about 250 abortions. Following interrogation, the Police Office arrested thirty-two-year-old Yamaguchi Naka and some others for the same crime.[58] The example suggests that *mumenkyo-sanba*, as old members of the community, were more inclined to agree to the requests of their clients than implement the regulations of the remote central government.

In contrast to the traditional practitioners, *shin-sanba* were, in principle, opposed to the practice of abortion and infanticide. The Meiji nation, conscious of the need for human capital to achieve successful modernization, regarded reproduction as a priority issue. In this milieu, officials assigned a role to new-midwives, which involved their interaction with both the authorities and lay women.[59] Officials formally required new-midwives to sign birth and death certificates and report illicit lay reproductive practices, thus contributing to the constant surveillance of lay people. This role of the new-midwives, as the instrument of the modern and legal, was a direct challenge to lay pre-modern expectations, assumptions and demands. As a result, the new-midwives often faced a quandary in practice, the more loyal they were to the national mission in their professional activity, the less popular they became in the eyes of clients and the more likely they were to be excluded from the medical market controlled by clients and *kyû-sanba*.

OLD-MIDWIVES CRIMINALIZED

The modern birth attendants attacked the popular *mumenkyo-sanba* from the 1870s through to the first decade of the twentieth century, exactly the period when *kyû-sanba* were stigmatized in *Josan no Shiori*. The journal publicized the arrests of *mumenkyo-sanba* in two sections: *zatsuroku* (miscellaneous records) or *zappô* (miscellaneous reports). The April 1912 issue reported that Izumi Jû, a 'fifty-eight-year-old unlicensed old woman from the City of Sakai [a suburb of the city of Osaka] was prosecuted for the second time on 17 November 1911 for her [continued] midwifery practice, after previously being ordered to pay a fine of five yen'.[60] Another report of May 1900 stated 'on the third of the last month, the Police Office prosecuted an old woman called Mrs Shiokawa from Nakamichi, Nakamoto-Village, who was found to have practised midwifery without a license'.[61] The journal re-emphasized the image of the monstrous illegal *mumenkyo-sanba*. Under the title 'Punishment of An Evil Midwife', the April 1900 issue reported that a *mumenkyo-sanba* in Kisarazu was sentenced to a nine-year term of imprisonment because she suffocated an infant and buried it near the family's outdoor toilet.[62] The article concluded: '. . . it is a bad event that evokes shuddering. The act by the non-licensed midwife is akin to the evil that an ogre does'.[63]

The journal considered these criminal *mumenkyo-sanba* deserved to be publicly shamed. The sixth issue of *Josan no Shiori* (November 1896) included short news items in the *zappô* section. With a bold title, it reported:

Punishment of an unlicensed midwife

Two unlicensed midwives from the city of Osaka, who openly practised unlicensed midwifery and misled ignorant people, were arrested and prosecuted by the authorities. We must celebrate this victory for those who practise midwifery after passing an approved midwifery examination.[64]

In addition, *Josan no Shiori* published the personal details of those who were convicted in order to make their exposé more telling. The June 1919 issue, for instance, gave all the personal details of the criminals:

Private midwives punished

Below are those against whom Police Offices brought a supplementary suit on March 4 of this year, for their conduct of private midwifery:

Yamase Sen (71)   187 Tsukuda, Senfuna-Village, Nishinari-Gun, Osaka
Kitamura Yoshi (52) 7, Kita 5-Chome, Denpo-Town, Nishinari-Gun, Osaka
Ueno Kiku (55)   27, Kita 2-Chome, Denpo-Town, Nishinari-Gun, Osaka
Kitano Riu   312 Shikanshima-Cho, West-Ward, Osaka-City.[65]

Clearly, the condemnation of *mumenkyo-sanba* had a purpose, which was to do with the professional reputation and role of midwives. The April 1899 issue of the journal told of a *mumenkyo-sanba*, Mrs Yamaguchi from Kanagawa, who was prosecuted, fined and sentenced to penal servitude for murdering both a mother and her infant.[66] Such incidents, the report concluded, 'not only harm mother and infant but also harm the reputation of new-midwives'.[67]

Although *shin-sanba* (and modern obstetrician–gynaecologists) drew a clear-cut line between themselves and *kyû-sanba* and *mumenkyo-sanba*, they also acknowledged that their clients did not share the same view. For lay people, all were *sanba* and belonged to the same category. The journal chose to shame illicit midwives and encourage *shin-sanba* to support the actions and policies of the authorities and watch out for dangerous and anti-modern *sanba*.

Other groups shamed

Shame tactics were also employed by the journal to challenge other groups who had flirted with illicit practices. *Josan no Shiori* ruthlessly attacked clients who not only committed a criminal act but also befriended *mumenkyo-sanba*. The October 1911 issue reported this news:

Umemoto Tome from Amagasaki, Hyogo (46) was fined five yen last May for working as a midwife without a license. Later Amagasaki Police Office found that she had practised abortion on the night of 1 July on Hana (31), the wife of Tsukino Yotarô from Ôsu-Village of Amagasaki, and that she had practised midwifery on the third of last month on the wife of Kaji Kyûgorô from Daimotsu-Village, Shima (25). Having interrogated her, the Police Office sent the documents to the public prosecutor on the thirteenth.[68]

Shin-sanba themselves were not exempt from shaming if they became involved in illicit practices. In the south ward of the city of Osaka, second-hand clothes trader, Nakai Yuku, was arrested for her illegal midwifery but the licensed midwives 'Hasegawa Toi (36), 866 Kanda-Town, Nanbahigashi, Osaka-City' and 'Yamanishi Tsune (30), Imamiyamura-Village, Nishinari-Gun, Osaka' were prosecuted for lending Nakai a license for fifty yen and an advertisement board for one yen per month.[69]

CONCLUSION

The articles in *Josan no Shiori* reflected the birth scene in Meiji Japan. Despite the efforts of the enlightened government and obstetrician–gynaecologists, who encouraged the training of new-midwives to change the local pre-modern birth culture, the free medical market that survived throughout the modern period ensured the survival of *kyû-sanba*, who remained popular not only because they were cheap to hire but also because they were familiar to their clients and open to their demands regarding abortion and infanticide.

Modern 'new-midwives' and obstetrician–gynaecologists were born out of the Meiji modernization scheme and thus were newcomers to the birth culture of Meiji Japan. Despite having the most advanced, and therefore supposedly the most effective, medical knowledge relating to midwifery and obstetrics, these practitioners did not readily assume the general management of pregnancy and birth. Lay clients regarded these modern birth attendants as expensive and only to be employed in case of complications, they preferred to rely on *kyû-sanba* in the first instance. Moreover, some feared the 'new-midwives' and modern obstetrician–gynaecologists for their role as reproductive police in the community. Thus, *shin-sanba* were confronted by a dilemma; their professionalism demanded they adhere to the national regulations but the reality in practice was that illegal abortion and infanticide persisted as a traditional practice and a necessary evil.

As a result, *shin-sanba* employed several tactics to promote themselves to the public. Some appeased the modernized *kyû-sanba* in the hope of obtaining referrals from them, whereas others learned local knowledge from *toriagebaba* to familiarize themselves with the local birth culture. Consequently, the practice of *shin-sanba* in the field grew out of their negotiation with several different actors: the modern obstetrician–gynaecologists, the local representatives of state authority, 'old-midwives' and, above all, their clients.

Josan no Shiori continually polemicized against this reality. In case histories, new-midwives reified the dichotomous formula of dangerous and illicit *kyû-sanba* versus safe and legitimate *shin-sanba* by reiterating stories where the *kyû-sanba* caused problems and *shin-sanba* rectified them. At the same time, *shin-sanba* ridiculed whoever remained 'pre-modern' or flirted with such elements. In this context, the construction of sinister *kyû-sanba* and ignorant clients helped to forge solidarity among modern birth attendants against the scapegoat, the 'pre-modern'. In taking this stand, authors included the national population rhetoric in their writing. Medical birth attendants, the products of the modern nation, stressed their superiority over *kyû-sanba* by emphasizing what they possessed and their opponents did not have, i.e. Western medical knowledge and support from the government.

From 1900, the needs of modern warfare favoured modern medical practitioners. Medical birth attendants were assigned responsibility for strengthening the national physique by delivering healthy babies who were to become strong soldiers and mothers for future generations. In addition, the emergence of a new middle class, the preferences of professional women, and the middle-class democratic movements of the twentieth century all popularized medical midwives in urban areas. Women's magazines, the products of a new media culture, hailed the professional medical midwives. From the 1920s, *shin-sanba* had won the race and become the dominant birth attendants. By then, the client family, familiar with scientific childbirth from the new media, craved *shin-sanba*'s medical care.[70] By the mid-1920s, the campaign waged by *Josan no Shiori* against the *kyû-sanba* ceased.

NOTES

1 For the modernization of Japan since the Meiji period, see for instance, C. Gluck, *Japan's Modern Myths*, Princeton: Princeton University Press, 1985 and Masao Maruyama, *Thought and Behaviour in Modern Japanese Politics*, Oxford: Oxford University Press, 1963.

2 British midwives were not subject to regulation and examination until the early twentieth century. For the historiography of handywomen, see L. Marks, *Model Mothers: Jewish Mothers and Maternity Provision in East London, 1870*, Oxford: Clarendon Press, 1994; several chapters in H. Marland and A. M. Rafferty (eds), *Midwives, Society and Childbirth: Debates and Controversies in the Modern Period*, London: Routledge, 1997; and H. Marland (ed.), *The Art of Midwifery: Early Modern Midwives in Europe*, London: Routledge, 1993; and the classic J. Donnison, *Midwives and Medical Men: a History of Inter-professional Rivalries and Women's Rights*, London: Heinemann, 1977.

3 In some regions, midwifery was considered to be an ignoble profession as practitioners inevitably touched the culturally inscribed *kegare* (impurities) such as blood and/or death. See B. Steger, 'From impurity to hygiene: the role of midwives in the modernization of Japan', *Japan Forum*, 1994, Vol. 6, pp. 175–87, and M. Nishikawa, *Aru Kindai Sanba no Monogatari: Noto, Takeshima Mii no Katari yori*, Tokyo: Midori no Yakata, 1989. For call-out and referral practices in early-modern Britain, see A. Wilson, *The Making of Man-midwifery: Childbirth in England 1660–1770*, London: UCL Press, 1995.

4 For a discussion of Japanese eugenics, see S. Otsubo and J. R. Bartholomew, 'Eugenics in Japan: some ironies of modernity, 1883–1945', *Science in Context*, 1998, Vol. 11, pp. 545–65.

5 See Onshi Zaidan Aiikukai (ed.), *Nihon San'iku Shuzoku Shiryô Shûsei*, Tokyo: Daiichi Hoki Shuppan, 1977.

6 M. Ogata, *Nihon Sankagaku-shi*, Tokyo: Maruzen: 1919, p. 426.

7 M. Ogata, *Saiyûki*, Kanehara Shôten, 1910.

8 Osakashi Sanbakai (ed.), *Osaka-shi Sanba Dantaishi*, Osaka: 1935.

9 M. Ogata, *Nihon Sankagaku-shi*, pp. 427–8. He and his followers also wrote articles for *Josan no Shiori*. The term *josanpu* was officially recognized after the Second World War, in 1947.

10 N. Naito, Y. Akai, and F. Higuma, 'Kako kara Mirai eno Apurôchi (1)', *Josanpu Zasshi*, 1997, Vol. 51(4), pp. 61–5.

11 M. Ogata, 'Josanpu no Kairyo ni Tsuite', *Josan no Shiori*, June 1896, p. 1.

12 The concept of dichotomous 'normal' and 'abnormal' childbirth emerged in Japan only during the late Meiji period, in association with the new knowledge of modern birth attendants. See A. Homei, '"Normal birth" and "modern hygiene": politics surrounding modern midwife's expertise', *The Japanese Journal of the History of Biology*, Vol. 70, forthcoming. See also E. Shorter, 'The management of normal deliveries and the generation of William Hunter,' in: W. F. Bynum and R. Porter (eds), *William Hunter and the Eighteenth-century Medical World*, Cambridge: Cambridge University Press, 1985, pp. 371–83.

13 In present Japanese, *jikken* primarily means 'experiment'.

14 M. Morita, 'Sokui Bunben no Ni-jikken,' *Josan no Shiori*, October 1910, (65), pp. 278–80.

15 Ibid., p. 278.

16 Ibid., p. 278.

17 Ibid., p. 279.

18 T. Matsuyama, 'Ein Haretsu ni Inbu Fushu wo Heihatsu Shitaru Ichi-jikken,' *Josan no Shiori*, November 1896, (6), pp. 196–7.

19 Ibid., p. 196.

20 Ibid., p. 197.

21 Ibid.

22 Ibid.

23 For the framework, see R. Porter (ed.), *Patients and Practitioners: Lay Perceptions of Medicine in Pre-industrial Society*, Cambridge: Cambridge University Press, 1985.

24 M. Morita, 'Zenchi Taiban no Ichi-jikken,' *Josan no Shiori*, September 1899 (40), pp. 226–7.

25 Ibid., p. 226.

26 Ibid., p. 227.

27 K. Yoshida, 'Bôsô Ninshin no Ichirei – Kyû-sanba no Goshin – Josanpu Shoshi ni Nozomu,' *Josan no Shiori*, August 1899 (39), p. 202.

28 Shingorô Takahashi, 'Chihô Kaigyô Josanpu ni Hojohi wo Kyûsuru no Hitsuyô,' *Josan no Shiori*, June 1909, (157), p. 2942.

29 S. Ishizaki, 'Meiji-ki no Seishoku wo Meguru Kokka Seisaku,' *Rekishi Hyoron*, April 2000, (600), pp. 39–57. For international comparisons and statistics, see also I. Loudon, *Death in Childbirth: an International Study of Maternal Care and Maternal Mortality*, Oxford: Clarendon Press, 1992.

30 T. Kawakami, *Gendai Nihon Irôshi*, Tokyo: Keiso Shobo, 1990, and Y. Kawakita, *Kindai Igaku no Shiteki Kiban*, Tokyo: Iwanami Shoten, 1977.

31 Kawakami: *Gendai Nihon Irôshi*.

32 Novels by Kazuharu Shima illustrate this point. Although semi-fictional in style, they are extremely revealing as they describe in detail the lives of *shin-sanba* during the Taisho and Showa periods. Kazuharu Shima, *Ichiman-nin no Ubugoe wo Ki'ita*, Tokyo: Shinchosha, 1986, and Kazuharu Shima, *Ubugoya no Onna Tachi*, Tokyo: Kenyukan, 1981.

33 For instance, the new-midwife Kobaru Fumi, who came from a mountainous remote area of Miyazaki Prefecture, recalled that her clients sometimes made fun of her skills because she was 'young'. Interview between Kobaru Fumi and the author, October 1999, Miyazaki, Japan.

34 H. Kobayashi, 'Shôsoku,' *Josan no Shiori*, March 1913 (202), pp. 1162–3.

35 For the construction of 'modernity' in modern Japan, see, for instance, S. Vlastos (ed.), *Mirror of Modernity: Invented Traditions of Modern Japan*, Berkeley: University of California Press, 1998. See also, for the construction of the 'Japanese people' during the modern time, E. Oguma, *Nihonjin no Kyôkai*, Tokyo: Shinyosha, 1998.

36   N. Yoshimura, *Kodomo wo Umu*, Tokyo: Iwanami Shoten, 1996. Also, as an example, see R. Kido, *Sanba Tebikigusa*, Fukuoka-ken Eiseika, 1896.

37   Cited after H. Hasegawa, 'Byôinka' Izen no Osan: Kumano deno Kikitori Chôsa yori,' *Shiso*, 1993, (824), p. 72.

38   Shima: *Ichiman-nin no*, and *Ubugoya no*.

39   Urashima, 'Awarenaru Boji', *Josan no Shiori*, May 1904, (96), p. 1107.

40   Y. Ikegami, '37-nen Nikki no Ichi', *Josan no Shiori*, April 1905 (107), pp. 1415–16.

41   Ikegami: April 1905, p. 1416.

42   T. Ueda, 'Hantô-ji no Ichirei', *Josan no Shiori*, April 1905 (107), pp. 1410–12.

43   Interestingly, it is believed that the founder of Tenri-kyô was a midwife, Miki. See H. Hardacre, *Marketing the Menacing Fetus in Japan*, Berkeley: University of California Press, 1997, pp. 19–54.

44   K. Takagaki, 'Santai Bunben no Ichirei', *Josan no Shiori*, July 1899 (38), pp. 171–5.

45   Ibid., pp. 171–2.

46   Ibid., p. 172.

47   S. Garon, *Molding Japanese Minds: the State in Everyday Life*, Princeton: Princeton University Press, 1998.

48   Women's magazines that flourished from this period onwards contributed to normalizing married adults with children.

49   Hardacre, *Marketing the Fetus*, and W. R. LaFleur, *Liquid Life: Abortion and Buddhism in Japan*, Princeton: Princeton University Press, 1992.

50   See, for instance, M. Tanitabe, 'Akago Yôiku Shihô ni tsuite', in Sôgô Joseishj Kenkyûkai (ed.), *Sei to Shintai*, Tokyo: Yoshikawa Kobunkan, 1998, pp. 327–61; M. Sawayama, *Shussan to Shintai no Kinsei*, Tokyo: Keiso Shobo, 1998; Yuki Sakurai, 'Mabiki to Datai', in *Nihon no Kinsei,* Vol. 15, Tokyo: Chuo Koronsha, 1993, pp. 97–128.

51   M. Sawayama, *Shussan to (Childbirth and body in the pre-modern)*, Tokyo: Keisô Shobô, 1998. Sawayama excellently demonstrated farmers' 'mentality' in the act of abortion. She challenges historians who presumed that Edo farmers possessed no empathy towards infants, enabling them to commit infanticide.

52   S. Burns, 'Between national policy and local practice: reproductive crimes in early Meiji Japan', Conference Presentation at the Twelfth Berkshire Conference on the History of Women, June 2002.

53   See Y. Fujime, *Sei no Rekishi-gaku*, Tokyo: Fuji Shuppan, 1998; and Shoko Ishizaki, 'Nihon no Dataizai no Seiritsu,' *Rekishi Hyoron*, 1997 (571), pp. 53–70.

54   Cited by Burns, 'National policy and local practice'.

55   'Onibaba no Datai,' *Josan no Shiori*, July 1912 (194), p. 838.

56   Weimer Germany interestingly manifested a striking similarity on this point. See C. Usborne, *The Politics of the Body in Weimer Germany: Women's Reproductive Rights and Duties*, Hampshire: Macmillan, 1992.

57   'Odorokubeki Aku-Sanba,' *Josan no Shiori*, November 1911 (186), p. 472.

58   Ibid.

59   Y. Terazawa, Gender, knowledge, and power: reproductive medicine in Japan, 1790–1930, PhD Dissertation, Los Angeles: University of California, Los Angeles, 2001.

60   'Mumenkyo-sanba,' *Josan no Shiori*, April 1912 (191), p. 703.

61   'Mumenkyo-sanba no Kokuhatsu,' *Josan no Shiori*, May 1900 (48), p. 119.

62   'Akusanba no Shobatsu,' *Josan no Shiori*, April 1900 (47), pp. 93–4.

63   Ibid., p. 94.

64   'Mumenkyo-sanba no Shobatsu,' *Josan no Shiori*, November 1896 (6), p. 209. Emphasis in the original.

65   'Shi'i-sanba Shobatsu,' *Josan no Shiori*, June 1919 (277), p. 4415.

66   'Mumenkyo-sanba no Shobatsu': April 1899 (113).

67 Ibid.
68 'Mumenkyo-sanba Futakumi,' *Josan no Shiori*, October 1911 (185), p. 440.
69 'Otafuku no Kanban,' *Josan no Shiori*, January 1913 (200), p. 2080.
70 See Terazawa, *Gender, Knowledge, Power*. In the remote areas where only a few physicians were available, the three-layered system persisted longer.

6 US organized medicine's perspective of nursing

Review of the *Journal of the American Medical Association*, 1883–1935

Brigid Lusk and Julie Fisher Robertson

Nursing and medicine are inexorably intertwined, through a shared interest in patient welfare. This professional proximity has encouraged members of both groups to observe and respond to the activities of the other. Following the introduction of formal nurse preparation in the US during the 1870s, there is evidence that physicians welcomed the presence of educated nurses at their side. The early records of the Illinois Training School for Nurses cite several instances of physician approbation of trained nursing care. For example, in 1882 a Cook County surgeon wrote:

> A week ago, standing by the bedside of a little boy, a victim of that dread disease hydrophobia, I could not help admiring the tender care which rendered his last hours more bearable. No mother could have done half so much for her own child as this nurse did for her charge, and in the face of risking her own life by so doing.[1]

Yet later physicians wrote scathingly of the education of nurses and their perceived encroachment upon medical practice. For example, a 1928 editorial in the *Illinois Medical Journal* discussed the 'presumptuous, physician-dominating, over-trained, dictatorial nurses and their mock practice of medicine'.[2]

In this chapter, we examine and analyse the development of this attitudinal change through nursing-related literature that appeared in the *Journal of the American Medical Association* (*JAMA*) from 1883 to 1935. This time period was pivotal for the development of both professions. A description of the changing fortunes of nursing and medicine is included to provide necessary contextual information. While medicine was transforming itself into a scientific profession, nursing – conceived as a respectable new field for women – struggled with inferior training schools and limited career prospects. Historical data show that nursing was significantly shaped by the paternalistic dominance of medicine, with its overpowering forces of gender and social class.[3]

JAMA first appeared as the weekly publication of the American Medical Association (AMA) in July 1883. It was modelled on the successful *British Medical Journal*, which had produced positive benefits for the British Medical Association in terms of membership and revenues.[4] The new journal was a success. In 1875, the AMA's membership totalled just over 1,400 and by 1885 membership had grown to almost 4,000. In 1930, about 100,000 of the nation's 125,000 practising physicians were AMA members, who regularly received their weekly copies of *JAMA*.[5] Nathan S. Davis, the venerable physician responsible for founding the AMA in 1847, was the journal's first editor.

JAMA presents a singularly appropriate source for this study. Most mainstream or regular physicians who had been educated in traditional, scientifically based colleges were members of the AMA and read its journal. The various medical sects or irregulars, such as homeopaths, hydropaths and eclectics, had enjoyed a strong following in the nineteenth century, but by the turn of the twentieth century regular physicians increasingly dominated US medicine. Regular physicians also were overwhelmingly male, because women were rarely accepted at good regular medical colleges. Women instead studied at the irregular medical colleges or small regular colleges, many of which were closed during the medical education reforms following the 1910 Carnegie Foundation Report. Moreover, women were not officially accepted as AMA members until 1915, although some state medical societies did allow female membership. [6] Thus, *JAMA* readers and contributors overwhelmingly represented the professionally powerful and male-dominated stronghold of the majority of US medical practitioners.

For this study, we reviewed all issues of *JAMA* from 1883 to the mid-Depression year of 1935, seeking references to nursing. The study concluded at 1935 because there was a reduction in *JAMA*'s public comments on nursing as a result of an increased focus on the issue of socialized medicine. The data surveyed included articles, editorials, news items, book reviews and correspondence. Editorials and editorial comments were unsigned and could have originated with any of the several editorial contributors. In addition, *JAMA* content related to medical professionalism and medical economics was reviewed to provide contextual depth. Secondary sources included histories of nursing and medicine as well as contemporary published literature.

Because nursing was, and remains, affected by medicine's assessment of its activities, *JAMA*'s early articles offer an opportunity to trace the evolution of interprofessional relationships from a medical viewpoint. Further, this study provides insight into contemporary gender relations, as nursing quickly became predominantly female; by contrast, the number of women physicians – never large – declined dramatically during the period studied. Thus, societal mores concerning gender roles, the rise of feminism in the 1890s and the delay in the enfranchisement of women form part of the background to this study.

The period from 1883 to 1935 includes the period of progressive-era initiatives, when reformers tried to address the ills of industrialization and urbanization; the Spanish–American War; the First World War; the influenza pandemic and the Great Depression. During this period, the fortunes of the medical profession in the US soared, while the professional and economic aspirations of nurses fell. By 1935, concerns about the cost of medical care and the threat of some form of socialized medicine consumed the interests of the nation's doctors to the virtual exclusion of what had become known as the 'nursing problem'.

HONEYMOON PERIOD FOR NURSING

The first mention of trained nursing in *JAMA* appeared in October 1883 when the editor, Dr Nathan S. Davis, reported on two resolutions adopted at a recent meeting of the AMA in Cleveland. These were:

> Whereas, good nursing is of paramount importance to the comfort of the sick and the restoration of their health, and
>
> Whereas, the subject is one which strongly addresses itself to the common sense and kindly sympathy of every intelligent member of society, therefore,
>
> Resolved, that this Association, fully recognizing the importance of the subject, respectfully recommend the establishment in every country town in our states and territories, of schools or societies for the efficient training of nurses, male and female, by lectures and practical instruction, to be given by competent medical men, members, if possible, of county societies, either gratuitously or at such reasonable rates as shall not debar the poor from availing themselves of their benefit.[7]

Nurse training schools had been established in several large US cities following the opening of the first nurse training schools in the 1870s. However, these schools were limited in number. Physicians, under the auspices of the local medical societies, were urged to become personally involved in nursing education to prepare adequate numbers of nurses for rural districts and villages. Nathan Davis' October 1883 editorial quoted a Dr Gross, who said: nursing 'can not fail to be instrumental in saving many lives, in preventing much suffering, [and] in inspiring hope in the sick.'[8]

JAMA's early contributors apparently held trained nurses in esteem. In 1883, a Michigan doctor claimed: 'At the present time it is evident that the country requires more nurses, and less doctors, more training schools for nurses, and less diploma mills for grinding out doctors'.[9] An 1888 editorial noted 'to undertake any argument as to the value of trained nurses at the present day would be scarcely less than a reflection on the intelligence of the reader'.[10] New training schools were noted with enthusiasm and extensive education was considered necessary. This editorial continued:

> There need be no fear that the nurse will know too much; that she never can. It need not be feared that if she knows a great deal she will be meddlesome; only the ignorant are meddlers, and the denser the ignorance the more and worse the meddling.[11]

Commencement addresses and annual reports of nurse training schools were sometimes noted in *JAMA*, and these were highly complimentary of the concept of nurse training and the character of the nurses. In 1885, an address to nurses who had just completed their training at a New York charity hospital asserted:

Among the nurses now may be found many ladies of culture and refinement and the skill of the physician has been supplemented by the skill of the educated nurse. The care and sympathy received by the patients promoted their recovery; while the presence among them of the pupils of the school so improved the moral tone of the institution that the cells for punishment were no longer necessary, and were removed. The death rate of the Hospital has steadily diminished since the introduction of the training school . . . it is now nearly 60 per cent less than before the establishment of the school, [as a result of] the increased efficiency in nursing, due to the careful training of intelligent nurses.[12]

During an AMA meeting of May 1888, the Visiting Nurse Society of Philadelphia was described. Supported by voluntary contributions, the nurses cared for those unable to afford skilled care. A physician noted:

I have known these nurses to go in an attic or cellar in the heart of the slums of the city, the rooms reeking with filth and overrun with vermin. The patients, fit inhabitants of their homes, destitute of the bare necessities of life, not having even a receptacle in which to boil water . . . In a few hours the nurses have cleaned the room, supplied the necessary furniture and utensils and prepared the patient for an abdominal section. With such an organization at his command, the physician has no reason to fear undertaking any case, surgical or medical, at the homes of even the poorest of patients.[13]

That same year, in a *JAMA* editorial describing the successes of the Illinois Training School for Nurses, Chicago, the efforts to obtain funding for nursing the sick poor were enumerated.[14]

During the last years of the nineteenth century, while nursing was attracting such approving comments from physicians, the US medical profession was struggling with the varied and unregulated nature of medical education and low professional self-esteem. 'Regular'[15] physicians received about the same low level of societal approval as the 'irregulars' – homeopaths, eclectics and others. In 1883, Davis, the editor of *JAMA*, printed an address he had recently delivered concerning the present status of the medical profession, he noted: 'at the present time . . . it is apparent upon almost every page of our medical literature, and from the discussions in every medical society, that many things exist which are far from being satisfactory either as regards its [medicine's] legal standing and educational progress'. He described the country's '60 or 70 independent medical schools . . . far the larger number still adhering to four and five months repetitional courses of instruction annually, with only one examination at the close . . . each carefully avoids any positive increase in the actual requirements for graduation for fear that its rivals will not do the same'.[16]

In 1885 there were 128 medical schools in the US and Canada, 101 of them for 'regular' physicians. During the 1880s, *JAMA* commentary decried professional overcrowding:[17]

Perhaps on no other subject is there greater unanimity of opinion among members of the medical profession, than that we have in this country too many medical colleges from which are annually graduated a number of students largely in excess of the legitimate needs of the people, and thereby productive of all the evils of an overcrowded profession.[18]

A paper quoted a past AMA president as asserting, in 1888, that:

An almost universal inclination prevails among the working classes to become doctors and lawyers . . . energetic and quick-witted young men in the ranks of the working classes can, by becoming doctors and lawyers, gratify their desires with less exertion than they would be compelled to put forth in other pursuits.[19]

The following decade saw continued problems with medical professionalism. There were 132 medical schools in the US in 1893, of which just ninety-four were 'regular'.[20] Most of the schools gave three-year courses but few medical students had undergraduate degrees: one in twelve, compared to one in five lawyers. In 1891, the president of the University of Indiana, a medical man, stated: 'Of all classes of students those in medicine are, as a rule, the most reckless in their mode of life, and the most careless of the laws of hygiene and of decencies in general'.[21] Many editorials referred to the varied quality of medical education and as the nineteenth century came to an end, the medical profession remained in disarray while nurses were lauded and valued for their care of the sick. Yet the constant discontent about the country's medical education found in the pages of *JAMA* during the 1880s revealed a unity of purpose among medical men that boded well for future professional action.

EMERGING CONCERNS ABOUT NURSING: THE 1890S

During the late 1890s, the pages of *JAMA* showed evidence of a decline in some physicians' appreciation of trained nursing and a developing wariness of nurses' professional aspirations. As the number of nurse training schools expanded and the presence of trained nurses became less novel, more physicians were exposed to the concept of educated women ministering to their patients. Outside the hospital, it might be expected that the feminist movement of the 1890s would negatively influence physicians' opinions of this new female occupation. However, an 1896 *JAMA* editorial rebutted a British medical article that was critical of over-ambitious and over-educated nurses, although the journal's support was tinged with gallantry rather than serious appreciation of the nurse's role:

We believe no American physician would for one moment deny that . . . the whole atmosphere of the ward and clinic is purified of the former vulgarity and rowdyishness by the silent presence of 'petticoats,' the white-capped priestesses of dignity and purity hovering about.[22]

The editor closed critically, asserting that women are 'good . . . [in] obeying, poor in leading' and that 'instances have been known in which the chief nurse has been an inexhaustible fountain of trouble and injustice . . . it would seem well not to allow too much autocratic power and authority to her ladyship'.[23]

Another editorial that appeared in 1899 discussed the new innovation of school nurses in London and summarized their duties. The editor's comment was approving if 'the nurses do not get too high an idea of their ability, and attempt to treat cases which belong to a physician'.[24] A book review from this period, one of several for nursing textbooks, also voiced a concern that perhaps nurses were overstepping the boundaries of nursing. The reviewer wrote: 'If any criticism is called for, it is that it goes into the subject of treatment . . . a little more fully than is necessary'.[25]

Later that same year, an editorial referred to a case in which a sponge had been left in a patient's abdomen following surgery. The nurse was found to be at fault because she was the person responsible for counting the sponges. *JAMA*'s comment was:

> The surgical nurse is a very important person in an operation, not possibly as important as she may sometimes think she is, but still one that has a very useful and responsible function to perform . . . If a little more stress were laid on this point in the addresses to training school graduates, at the expense perhaps of some of the conventional glorification of the nursing profession, it would be no loss.[26]

However, several excerpts from the various state medical society proceedings documented continued support for the value of nurses' work, with comments such as nursing is a 'science',[27] and:

> . . . the physician . . . knew the value of the trained nurse, understood the close and vital relation she held to his patient; how much her care and quick intelligence of the needs did to relieve his anxiety and promote the welfare of his patients . . . The untrained nurse, on the other hand, was meddlesome and dangerous'.[28]

These comments were augmented by patriotic fervour instigated by the Spanish–American War of 1898. The prestige of nursing was generally enhanced in time of war[29] and there were several comments in *JAMA* about bills before Congress and the Senate that would formally recognize positions for trained female nurses in the army, which included positions of authority for female nurses. However, a *JAMA* editorial comment termed these 'singular propositions'.[30] An article by Nicholas Senn, a Chicago surgeon who had been Chief of the Operating Staff with the Army during the war, cited the poor nursing care men received at the hands of the army corps of male nurses, 'hundreds of recently enlisted men had to be detailed for hospital duty and were placed in charge of the sick . . . It takes months of hard work to make a soldier; it takes a much longer time to make a good nurse'.[31] The hospital ships, an innovation of this war, employed trained female nurses, and Senn thought these women were wonderful, both for their educated knowledge and their womanly skills:

> Ask any of the sick soldiers who returned on any of these ships, and you will find him ready to praise and bless the female nurse under whose care he was placed on his return from the seat of war . . . Woman is a natural nurse, and nowhere does she appear grander or nobler than when she is administering to the sick and dying of an army in active warfare. The American woman, above those of any other nation, is peculiarly well fitted for such a post of duty.[32]

Later in 1899, a *JAMA* editorial was less positive about the role of trained nurses in the army. A military journal, quoted in the editorial, had asserted that the introduction of female nurses 'would involve "much expense, idleness, risk of friction, and a certain disquiet about immorality." '[33] *JAMA*'s editor noted that these:

> . . . views may shock some of the worshipers of the trained nurse, who be-lieve that 'ministering angels,' at least terrestrial ones, are exclusively of the female sex . . . in war, many emergencies and conditions where their physical disabilities and due consideration for their sex absolutely prohibit the nursing services of women . . . The question [of trained female nurses in the armed forces] may therefore be regarded as no longer an open one.[34]

Thus, at least in the pages of *JAMA*, any prestige nurses garnered from their war efforts was short-lived. In spite of the commendations of an experienced army surgeon such as Senn, *JAMA*'s editor sought to disqualify female nurses from army service.

The confusion about nurses evident from these discordant medical views re-flects the real dilemma these men experienced. For decades, the role of women had been equated with purity and goodness; women were the natural guardians of family life and morals. Thus, women had been effectively excluded from the com-petitive male world of business and power outside the home.[35] Initially, women as nurses were allowed to bask in the saintliness traditionally accorded women as homemakers. They were perceived, in Senn's words, as 'ministering angels', grand, and noble. Yet these ministering angels were entering the work force and even the war arena as trained women. Meanwhile, the medical men were carving out their own professional turf. Outbursts against nurses in *JAMA*, the doctors' professional voice, were almost inevitable.

THE EARLY TWENTIETH CENTURY: CONCERNS ABOUT NURSING INTENSIFY

For nursing and medicine, the early years of the twentieth century were decisive in terms of professional growth. The growing numbers of medical students and their non-standardized, often poor, education brought forth demands for reform from the medical leaders. In 1900 there were 166 medical colleges in the US, of which 133 were regular.[36] By 1909, the number was down to 144, of which 117 were regular.[37] In 1907, a *JAMA* editorial noted that medical education was still unsatisfactory, although progress had been made.[38] However, as one author noted, the 'low standard of the medical education of the USA, as compared with that in other countries', remained a cause for concern.[39]

In nursing, hospital administrators recognized that economic advantages accompanied the operation of a nurses' training school because student nurses were low-cost, relatively skilled workers; the numbers of these nursing schools expanded exponentially. Nurses looked to the legislature to ensure standards within nursing education and to protect the title of nurse through formal registration. However, as women they still did not have the vote and were unable to directly influence legislation.

During this early period when medical practitioners were attempting to limit access to medical education, references to nursing in *JAMA* noted several areas of disquiet. One concern was that the poor could not afford trained nursing care, another that nursing education was non-standardized. A particular concern was that nurses were losing their subservient position relative to physicians, and finally nurses were perceived to encroach upon medical terrain.

The expense of employing trained nurses was a recurring theme. Following three years working in hospital as a student, trained nurses expected to find employment as fee-charging private duty nurses. However, few patients could afford their fees.[40] To resolve this problem, several proposals were put forward for cheaper, less-trained or untrained attendants. One idea was for two levels of trained nurse, one who had graduated from a regular diploma programme and another who had received just six months' training.[41] A physician wrote of his six-month course to train, what he termed, domestic nurses.[42] However, as one physician put it, these ideas were 'deplored by graduate nurses'.[43] An editorial in 1909 claimed that 'the attending physician often had to forgo his fee in order that proper nursing may be had'. The editor suggested that the student nurse's last six months of training be in the form of free private duty nursing care, he closed with the observation 'the nursing profession can hardly be expected to be as altruistic as the medical profession, but something should be done'.[44]

This problem was a real one. Private duty nurses who worked in middle-class homes imposed the total burden of their salary on one household or client. Other professions charged for each consultation or were paid by an agency. In reply to a 1905 correspondent who asked about the ethics of gratuitous service among professionals, the *JAMA* editor commented, 'The nurse, however, is not expected to give free services, because her work usually takes all her time, while that of the physician is one item in a day's work'.[45]

As medical care and nursing became more complex, *JAMA* printed comments on the need to restrict nursing practice. A 1906 editorial reprinted maxims from another medical journal, which included the following:

Every attempt at initiative on the part of nurses . . . should be reproved by the physicians. The programs of nursing schools and the manuals employed should be limited strictly to the indispensable matters of instruction for those in their position, without going extensively into purely medical matters which might give them a false notion as to their duties and lead them to substitute themselves for the physician. The professional instruction of . . . nurses should be intrusted [sic] exclusively to the physicians, who only can judge what is necessary for them to know.[46]

The editor gave his opinion that 'These maxims should certainly be borne in mind by the physician who has dealings with the nurse . . . that she be not encouraged to take steps that are not in her province'.[47] A few years later, in 1911[48] and 1914,[49] more guidelines for nurses appeared in the pages of *JAMA*, some of which had originally been devised by the British Medical Association. These noted: 'Sometimes nurses give annoyance to medical men by usurping the functions of the physician, in criticizing treatment, and in other ways'.[50]

Several reviews of nursing texts in this period argued that much more information was included than the nurse needed to know, or should know. An exception was Isabel Hampton Robb's 1901 book, *Nursing Ethics*; on this occasion the reviewer noted: 'The nurse who follows the advice here given will not come under the condemnation which has been uttered by various physicians . . . and which, it must be said, often has a very good basis'.[51] Another editorial attempted to clarify what the term 'good nursing' meant. The editor was concerned that the lay public might be confused by this phrase and that they might interpret it literally. Physicians, he explained, knew that the phrase meant nursing care under the constant and watchful supervision of the doctor:

Undoubtedly . . . improved nursing conditions in our hospitals have greatly lessened the mortality from the specific infectious disease . . . but this is only so because of the constant, sedulous supervision of trained medical skill . . . The public must not be allowed to drift into error in the matter.[52]

Once again there were calls to restrict nurse education or train a lower grade of nurse for the less serious cases. Two reports about a symposium on the 'over-trained nurse' asserted that the nurse of 1906 was given 'too much theory and too little practice'. One speaker wanted a return to the 'old-fashioned nurse whose principal asset was her sympathy and proper equipment of character'.[53]

For many years, attempts to place the physician in complete charge of nursing education were discussed at society meetings and a variety of strategies were discussed in the journal. A contributor in 1901 made a case for the introduction of a formalized curriculum, with the students paying for their tuition.[54] In 1903, *JAMA* printed an abstract from another journal in which the physician author argued that preliminary nursing education should be placed in a more formal setting, outside the hospital, to allow students to study without the pressure of nursing duties.[55] Another author reasoned that nurses were not receiving too much education, but that their education needed more depth and organization.[56] The balance in the curriculum attracted critical comment; some complained that nurses were taught too much anatomy, physiology, pathology, bacteriology and chemistry: 'More time should be devoted to teaching nurses household work, cooking, ordering of supplies, cleaning of rooms etc . . . The nurse must realize that any honorable labor is within her duties'.[57] In 1910, a New York physician noted:

> In all the meetings of the nurses associations, supervisors associations, and hospital superintendents associations, a good deal of eloquence is expended in the interest of the nurse and the training school and of the hospital, overshadowing completely the practicing physician, who gives bread and butter to the majority of all graduate nurses.[58]

The journal reported that, in 1908, the American Hospital Association spent the entire afternoon session of the opening day on 'The problem of training nurses and the requirements and course of training'.[59]

The topic of registration for nurses was also noted as it passed through the legislatures of various states during this period, with occasional more extensive discussion. Registration would separate trained nurses from untrained women who presented themselves as nurses. Nurses who completed an approved nursing education and passed a state licensure examination could call themselves registered nurses and use the letters RN after their names. The *JAMA* editor was scathing in his comments concerning the North Carolina legislature that had passed an act for the examination and registration of nurses, but refused to pass a medical practice bill.[60] Nurses in Illinois, home state of the American Medical Association, had a particularly difficult experience in securing nurse registration legislation. M. Helena McMillan, President of the Illinois State Association of Graduate Nurses, explained Illinois nurses' views of a proposed registration bill in the pages of *JAMA*. McMillan reported that in response to a perceived nurse shortage, and to provide cheaper nursing care, the Illinois State Association proposed to recognize two grades of nurse, one with twelve months and one with twenty-seven months of training.[61] An accompanying response was printed from a physician representative of the American Hospital Association. The physician derided McMillan's letter: 'Not only is there a shortage of nurses, but there is a growing tendency on the part of the registered nurse to escape doing private duty or actual nursing'. With respect to the two grades of nurses, he commented:

> The slave was chained to the galley for life, but that was centuries ago. Can it be that we are returning to that age? Is it possible that the law is to be invoked to create a class, to keep a person to a particular work, and to prevent the person from doing anything else? No matter what the junior nurse's ambitions may be, no matter what her ability as a teacher, as a supervisor or as an executive may be; no matter what her aptitude for public health service may be . . . because the registered nurse does not care to nurse the sick, she has no right to say that others who wish to shall not nurse, nor has she any right to say that nursing shall be done only under her supervision.[62]

The nurses were thus confronted with a vexing problem – their poorest patients could not afford nursing care – yet nurse leaders such as McMillan were ridiculed when she addressed this issue. Meanwhile, *JAMA*'s contributors argued that less-trained nurses would be cheaper and thus accessible for almost all patients. In effect, curtailing nurses' education would protect the professional aspirations of medicine admirably. Nurses would be clearly doctors' assistants rather than semi-autonomous practitioners in their own right. Nurses would finally be compelled to acknowledge their station.

THE FIRST WORLD WAR

For medicine, the professional outlook around the First World War was positive. In 1910, the Carnegie Foundation for the Advancement of Teaching produced a major report on medical education; this had a profound influence on restricting the availability of medical education. Inferior medical schools were publicly noted, which resulted in scores of schools closing over the following decade. *JAMA* editorials approved of the report and scoffed at assertions that women and the poor might now be excluded from medical education, or that there would be a shortage of doctors for rural areas.[63] Medical education now became more expensive, more onerous, and less crowded.

For nursing the opposite occurred. The First World War and the influenza pandemic of 1918–19 produced an increased need for nurses and a continuing expansion in the number of nursing schools.[64] In 1913 there were about 1,100 training schools for nurses,[65] yet the problem of affordable nursing care continued to be noted in *JAMA*'s pages. Many physicians' comments were variations on the theme of training 'the average wage-earning girl, who can read and write and spell, in one year so that she will be worth $10 or $12 a week . . . as a nurse'.[66] The very real problems of a career in nursing were summarized in the following comments:

> Take bright girls, with good education and good common sense, and very few will take a three years course in nursing when they understand that, after spending those three years in training, the time of their service will be about 10 years, and that perhaps half of that time they will be idle, and consequently will have very little saved at the end of that period . . . It is only natural for bright girls to seek some other kind of business.[67]

Once again, in this period there were several calls for different grades of nursing that would allow the less acutely ill to hire less well-educated nurses. However, some physicians noted problems with this idea, Richard Olding Beard, a University of Minnesota medical professor, asked whether the poor would then always be forced to hire 'Class B' nurses even when they were critically ill. Beard's concerns were epitomized in a letter from a physician, who wrote that six-month training schools should be opened to produce obstetric nurses devoted 'to taking care of the working man's wife'.[68] Beard called for state boards of nursing, standardization of nursing education, and increased numbers of university-based schools of nursing.[69] Another *JAMA* physician author, J. B. Howland, supported the case for more education for nurses. In 1913 Howland emphasized the breadth of nursing practice, including district nursing; anti-tuberculosis work; work in infant welfare clinics and milk stations; social and welfare work in department stores, social service departments of hospitals and settlement houses; school nursing; and working as hospital superintendents and training school instructors. 'So much is expected of nurses', Howland continued, 'that more care must be taken with their education.' Instead of making the course shorter and lowering standards, as many schools were doing to attract students, Howland argued that an excellent education open only to well-prepared women would increase the number and calibre of nurses.[70] Five pieces appeared in *JAMA* between 1912 and 1919 that gave credit to the work nurses were doing and often cited improved health outcomes that resulted from these expanded roles.[71]

With the entry of the US into the First World War in 1917, the pages of *JAMA* gave publicity to the recently inaugurated Army School of Nursing and the Nursing Corps of the US Navy.[72] The journal also discussed the need for Red Cross nurses and an editorial in 1918 appealed for more Red Cross nurses, noting that:

> In recent years she [the nurse] has developed into more than a doctor's assistant; she has become an important, and in some respects a necessary, aid in carrying on the social work that has developed during the last decade or two . . . nurses are one of the great needs in winning the war, and that it is our duty as physicians to aid in supplying this need.[73]

Yet almost before the ink was dry on the Treaty of Versailles, a January 1919 *JAMA* editorial complained about nurses. It opened with:

> What is the matter with the trained nurse? A wave of harsh and resentful criticism of the professional nurse seems to be sweeping the country . . . in spite of her magnificent and sacrificial service in the Great War, she is not now viewed by large numbers of physicians . . . as a ministering angel of mercy . . .[74]

The piece continued in this vein, lamenting that her elementary education and her training was too long. Nurses needed to be 'a household helper not too proud to assist in the kitchen . . . let the nurse be a little less autocratic, a little less dictatorial'.[75] The response from the AMA members was unanimously supportive: 'It is true, every word of it,'[76] 'I want to congratulate you,'[77] nurses need less 'brain stuffing,'[78] 'Truer words were never spoken'.[79] One lengthy letter came from a physician who, although he essentially agreed with the editor's premise, asserted that the cure lay in 'a broader education, with less routine menial work, better home environment, and more inspiring and stimulating contacts'.[80] In essence, whereas physicians were achieving greater professional standing, the problems with nursing did not abate. Nursing care by trained nurses was expensive and many people could not afford it. Many physicians voiced concern over nurses' plight but others went back to the old plea for nurses to accept less training and work for less pay. In the pages of *JAMA*, the nurses' war service was apparently forgotten as the problems of expensive care and the length of their training resurfaced.

THE 1920s

By 1920, the position of medicine was further consolidated; the number of medical schools had declined to eighty-three, of which seventy-six required two or more years of college work before admission. A 1921 *JAMA* editorial claimed: 'The object sought has been attained and medical education in the USA is now equal to, if it does not surpass, that in any other country'.[81] As physicians were fewer in number and better educated, and as treatment became more sophisticated, the increased cost of medical care became a hotly debated issue.

In 1929, *JAMA*'s new editor, Dr Morris Fishbein, introduced some colourful invective in response to critics of the high cost of medical care; Fishbein accused them of 'yawping, sneering,' and 'comical lucubrations'. He went on to accuse the director of the Rosenwald Foundation of 'sarcasm, half-baked opinions, and sops to the multitude'. In his editorial Fishbein spoke of 'physicians who have given themselves to mankind',[82] he went on to point out that the cost of nursing was one of several factors driving up the price of medical care.

Meanwhile, the number of nurse training schools continued to grow. These schools had increased from fifteen in 1880 (when there were 100 medical schools) to 1,755 in 1920 and 2,155 in 1926 (compared with seventy-nine medical schools).[83] Yet, the pages of *JAMA* indicated a concern with a shortage of nurses during the early 1920s. This concern was demonstrated through general correspondence,[84] a report of a hospital conference that featured the nursing shortage[85] and a news item that reported a drive to increase the numbers of student nurses.[86]

In his 1924 address to the delegates, the AMA's president-elect discussed the high cost of nurses as a primary factor increasing medical costs and again called for less nursing education as the solution to the problem:

> The trained nurse for ordinary service has become inaccessible . . . There is a need for her [the trained nurse] but there is a much greater need for a very large number of trained nurses who will perform the simple duties of attendants for the sick. That is the great function of the trained nurse. The things she has to do are simple things. The work she has to do in ordinary service does not require a high school training nor three years of hospital training.[87]

Yet the AMA's president-elect also noted that nurses were not receiving an education throughout their three years of hospital training: 'The nurses themselves are by no means entirely responsible for the present situation. Much of the time in their training has been taken up [by] the common menial duties of housemaids in the hospital'.[88]

Two years later, a *JAMA* editorial was less sympathetic when nurses in Chicago refused to continue working twenty-four hour shifts as private duty nurses for hospital patients. The editor commented:

> The demand means that a person requiring continuous attendance must employ two nurses where formerly he paid only one. For at least five years there has been increasing uneasiness among the medical profession and the public over the changing attitude of the nurse toward her vocation and her labor . . . nurses are being trained in technical matters to a point at which dignity suffers when they are asked to undergo the tribulations of personal service.[89]

The following year, a letter to the editor that complained about poor private duty nursing care and yearned for the 'good old days' was published. 'In days gone by, when nurses were receiving one half the remuneration which is being given them today and were working twice as many hours, they prided themselves on the neatness and accuracy of their record sheets'.[90] In response to that letter, another physician wrote 'I believe the fault belongs to three causes: Lack of interest, no pride in registry, and too much money . . . Since the eight hour service in hospitals was inaugurated there has been more chance existing to pass the buck from one shift to another'.[91]

In 1920, as the influenza pandemic continued to strain all medical services, Chicago's Commissioner of Health wrote of a two-month nursing course his office had inaugurated, which had already graduated over 1,000 nurses who were willing to do housekeeping as well as nursing. He justified this with 'In its final analysis, nursing is nothing more nor less than housekeeping for the sick'. The curriculum was designed to avoid all mention of medical matters because 'There is no other place in the universe where a little knowledge is so truly a dangerous thing as in medicine. These women know that they know nothing about materia medica – at least we told them so often enough'.[92] Surgeon William J. Mayo wrote about 'The nurse question', noting that the 'high standard registered nurse is one of the greatest blessings of modern civilization'. But he thought that lesser trained nurses, 'The Fords . . . of the nursing world,' were also needed. He was puzzled by the attitudes of the nurses' organizations:

> If representatives of the nurses' union are approached on the subject of vocational training to develop a large number of young women for this important work they are indignant and call attention to the fact that standards are being raised for physicians, and they ask why should they lower theirs. In this connection it should be remembered that the physician is expected to care for rich and poor alike, and allow no one to suffer for lack of such care, regardless of his ability to pay for service. This is not and can never be the case with the registered trained nurse.[93]

An editorial from that issue commented on Mayo's article. The shortage of nurses was noted before the editor continued:

He [Mayo] emphasizes, as the Journal has done, the fact that a highly trained nurse is not necessary in the vast number of cases of ordinary illness . . . [quoting a recent commencement address] any bright girl can be taught in sixty days to take a temperature, pulse and respiration accurately, to prepare and administer invalid diet, to administer drugs in numerous ways, to give baths and fomentations, and attend to the personal wants of the invalid.[94]

Nurses themselves tried to address the cost of graduate nursing care through initiatives such as group and hourly nursing, and these efforts were reported in *JAMA*. Group nursing was designed for hospital patients who wanted the services of a private duty nurse. Nurses cared for several adjoining patients who then split the fee. In hourly nursing, private duty nurses spent a short period rather than a complete shift with their patients.[95]

The AMA, along with its various state societies, took an active interest in nursing education during the 1920s. In 1923, the AMA's Committee on Trained Nursing commented on the non-standardized status of nursing education and suggested that the AMA, in conjunction with the National League of Nursing Education, form a committee of physicians, nurses and an educator, to devise and implement a 28-month curriculum and initiate a subsidiary nursing service. A minority report, written by Richard Olding Beard, noted that this proposal 'will be unwelcome to the profession of nursing . . . The medical profession of today must realize . . . it is no longer in a position, if it ever possessed the right, to dictate its conditions'.[96] Regarding subsidiary nurses, the minority report noted:

An inferior type of semi-educated nurse may not be offered to large classes of people who . . . are economically disabled by sickness, without incurring a sense of social injustice . . . The corollary of the proposal would lie in the offer of a second hand doctor at a diminished fee . . . The ethical error of the proposal of the 'subnurse' lies not only at the point of nursing service; it lies at the heart of nursing education. The women are not to be found who . . . will be content with a reparation and a position inferior to that which another group of nurses receives and occupies.[97]

The AMA was undaunted by these considerations and still pressed for two grades of nursing education. In 1926, the AMA's Special Committee on Nursing Education was formed to address the 'great need throughout the country for a basic trained nurse',[98] this group proposed a two-year course after which the graduates could be 'trained or, if preferred, registered nurses'. In 1927, after further study, the committee recommended a twenty-eight-month standard course and the training of a lesser-educated subsidiary nurse; in addition they supported strategies such as group and hourly nursing. Overall, the report was sympathetic to nurses and nursing, noting that nurses problems reflected 'the economic evolution of a group of workers sincerely trying to render the best possible social service'.[99] The following year, 1927, the AMA speaker proposed complete AMA control of nursing when he declared: 'The AMA should, yea must, undertake its [the problem of nursing education and service] solution . . . We become negligent and shrink our responsibilities . . . if we delegate the task to others'.[100]

Several state medical society reports on the status of nursing were shared with *JAMA* readers in 1928; they reveal that major problems were still apparent in nursing. The Medical Society of the State of New York was in sympathy with nursing, citing the increase in the number of nurse training schools 'some of which seem to be conducted merely because they need the service of nurses'.[101] The Michigan State Medical Society was more critical:

> Pupil nurses today are younger and less considerate than formerly. This is shown in their noisiness . . . the mechanical performance of duties and their lessened humility when mistakes are made . . . One seldom finds a nurse now, it is said, who will help with housework 'in a pinch,' help get the children to school or do some of the cooking as her predecessor did . . . The committee believes that nurses are over-educated. The committee recognizes the following principles for endorsement by the State Medical Society:
>
> 1. Nurses are helpers and agents of physicians, not co-workers or colleagues.
> 2. Physicians should have a part in the direction of the training of nurses and in its limitations as should the hospitals which give the training.
> 3. The training of nurses should be simplified and the time of undergraduate training reduced to not more that two years.
> 4. The apprenticeship system must be maintained.[102]

Reviews of nursing texts were still published in *JAMA* and criticisms of the amount and level of content continued. The author of one book was complimented; her work was not 'the usual half-baked treatise which attempts to make . . . the average nurse into a specialist'.[103] However, in a 1927 review of the collected addresses of M. Adelaide Nutting, the first nursing professor in the USA, Nutting was criticized for her elitist views on nursing and her pleas for endowments for nurses education:

> There is no indication of any anxiety about the production of the latter [less-educated] sort of nurse in this book. There is need for blunt consideration of this unpleasant topic. Nurses are not physicians. They are not in a position of independent responsibility. In no offensive sense, most of them should be servants for the sick. There is little evidence in the nursing literature of a willingness to face this fact.[104]

A committee to study nursing and nursing education, undertaken by seven nursing, medical and hospital associations and known as the Grading Committee, was initiated in 1926. An AMA member and medical school dean, Dr William Darrach, was appointed chair. Results of the work of this committee, indicating a gross over-supply of nurses, were regularly shared in *JAMA*.[105]

Overall, the problems with nursing were extensively noted in the pages of *JAMA* during this period. Yet the burgeoning national outcry over the high cost of medical care also received attention. Fishbein's contention that nursing costs were partly responsible for these escalating medical expenses added urgency, in *JAMA*'s pages, to cut the expense of nursing care. One sure method, it seemed, was to reduce the length of nurses' education.

THE DEPRESSION YEARS

With the onset of the Great Depression, items related to the cost of medical care dominated the editorial and correspondence pages of *JAMA*. It was asserted that patients demanded hospital care because the new-found income of working wives 'must not be disturbed'. 'If the hospital is too expensive, someone will have to wait for his money; and it requires no PhD to guess who that somebody is going to be'.[106] Health insurance was proposed by some economists as the only way to equitably cover the cost of medical care.[107] One study funded by the Rosenwald Foundation found that physicians' fees accounted for about 25 per cent of people's medical expenditure, hospitals and clinics about 30 per cent, and medicines and medical supplies about 25 per cent. Yet medical insurance and any form of state-supported medical care were vigorously rejected in the pages of *JAMA*. The loss of physician autonomy and ability to set their own fees in European countries, especially England and Germany, were frequently noted. In a 1930 address, outgoing AMA president Malcolm Harris asserted:

> Medicine is being besieged on every side by forces that are constantly growing stronger and stronger, and unless some defensive effort is made to break the siege the profession must eventually capitulate and become socialized and become employees of the state.[108]

Incoming AMA president William Morgan urged AMA members to: 'forestall further encroachments on prerogatives which, by virtue of training and experience, belong to us as private citizens, members of an honored and honorable profession'.[109]

The Committee on the Costs of Medical Care released a landmark report two years later in 1932, following a five-year study. The committee recommended some form of health insurance as well as more group medical practice. While the AMA initially supported this committee and it worked out of the AMA's Chicago headquarters, the report was greeted scathingly in the pages of *JAMA*. Fishbein's editorial accused committee members of personal bias towards health insurance and stated that the result was a foregone conclusion. 'Knowing the composition of the Committee on the Costs of Medical Care, it is interesting to find the pet plans of many of its members so sweetly elaborated'. A minority report was also published. These committee members noted, in their dissent, 'the shortest road to the commercialization of the practice of medicine is through the supposedly rosy path of insurance'. Fishbein urged all members to oppose the majority report, stating it represented the forces of 'socialism and communism'.[110]

As economic concerns filled *JAMA*'s pages, there were fewer references to nursing, although the 1934 final report of the grading committee was discussed. A *JAMA* review of the Grading Committee's final report, however, contested the committee's recommendation that nurses needed better education for their increasingly responsible positions because 'the evidence on which it is based is nowhere disclosed'.[111] Reflecting this, the editor noted: 'Opinions as to the proper function of the nurse are so divergent that these conclusions will not meet with unquestioning assent'.[112]

CONCLUSION

This chapter set out to demonstrate the complexity and interdependent nature of early professional relations between nursing and medicine. Initially, doctors were supportive of the new occupation of nursing. The women gave dignity and order to the wards, demonstrated positive health outcomes among the poor, and possibly enhanced medicine's self-esteem as doctors worked besides gracious and subordinate young women. But as the number of nurses increased while physicians became more rarefied, medicine's opinion of nursing changed.

The impact of gender in this discussion should be noted. As stated earlier, the AMA was closed to women until 1915 and, as far as could be discerned from their names, all the physicians identified in this review were male. When most of the irregular schools and small medical schools shut down during the early years of the twentieth century, medicine was essentially closed to women. Conversely, nursing was predominantly female. Thus, the journal reflects male physicians discussing female nurses – a scenario fraught with traditional imbalances of power.

Comments showing dismay with nurses in the early twentieth century might reflect a decrease in the quality and dedication of nurses. As the number of nursing schools increased, entrance standards were relaxed, especially as women were attracted to other work opportunities. Predominantly, it was organized medicine that sought to remedy the situation by declaring nursing a low-level skill. Medical control of nursing education was sought, with the intent of decreasing nurses' training and limiting nurses' knowledge. Even so, there were a minority of physicians who felt that problems with nursing were caused by nurses' inadequate education and wanted to raise entrance standards and educational quality. Unfortunately, these ideas were not implemented.

Throughout this period, 'regular' physicians were concerned with their own professional development as a learned body. This chapter has illustrated the frank self-interest of many members of the medical group. They sought to decrease the number of medical schools while increasing the quality of medical education. Overall, the view constructed from their own journal broadly interprets nursing in two ways, either as a potential threat to the medical profession (in much the same way as the 'irregulars') or as adjuncts to their professional authority. The doctors quoted in *JAMA*'s pages appeared supportive of nurses when they acted as women

– supporting and enhancing the traditional male medical role while embracing the nurturing, domestic role of nursing. These medical men slipped into a more critical stance when nurses attempted to attain their own professional identity and autonomy.

The debate about the nursing problem receded as the forces of the Great Depression initiated a campaign by organized medicine against the proponents of health insurance and socialistic medicine. This threat solidified organized medicine, as portrayed in the pages of *JAMA*, and moved the discourse away from interdisciplinary rivalries with nursing.

NOTES

1   G. F. Schryver, *A History of the Illinois Training School for Nurses 1880–1929*, Chicago: Chicago Board of Directors, 1930, pp. 35–6.
2   'Editorial: The nursing situation seen from many viewpoints', *Illinois Medical Journal*, 1928, Vol. 53, pp. 13–14.
3   See J. A. Ashley, *Hospitals, Paternalism, and the Role of the Nurse*, New York: Teachers College Press, Columbia University, 1976, and B. Melosh, *The Physician's Hand*, Philadelphia: Temple University Press, 1982. Both authors describe the complex interrelationship underlying the professional aspirations of nursing and medicine, and the impact of gender and social class that worked to support medicine's professional claims. See also C. Rosenberg's essay 'Healing hands: nursing in the hospital', in *The Care of Strangers. The Rise of America's Hospital System,* New York: Basic Books, 1987, pp. 212–36, Rosenberg wrote that the 'relationship between nursing and medicine was particularly problematic. Yet the fortunes of the two groups were indissolubly related; . . . the nature of their relationship presumed the subordination of nursing', p. 231.
4   M. Fishbein, *History of the American Medical Association*, Philadelphia: Saunders, 1947, p. 101.
5   M. Fishbein, 'Function and future of the AMA in medical education', *JAMA*, 1930, Vol. 94, pp. 911–15.
6   R. M. Morantz, 'The "Connecting Link": the case for the woman doctor in nineteenth-century America', in J. W. Leavitt and R. L. Numbers (eds), *Sickness and Health in America*, 3rd edn, Madison: University of Wisconsin Press, 1997, pp. 161–72; V. G. Drachman, 'Female solidarity and professional success: the dilemma of women doctors in late nineteenth-century America', in J. W. Leavitt and R. L. Numbers (eds), *Sickness and Health in America*, pp. 173–82; B. Lusk, 'Monstrous productions or the best of womanhood? Progressive-Era women in medicine', *Chicago History*, 2000, Vol. 28, pp. 4–21.
7   'Trained nurses', *JAMA*, 1883, Vol. 1 (9), pp. 430–1.
8   Ibid., p. 431.
9   J. F. Jenkins, 'Letter to the Editor: trained nurses for the country', *JAMA*, 1883, Vol. 1 (17), pp. 515–16.
10 'Trained nurses in the country', *JAMA*, 1888, Vol. 11, pp. 311–12.
11 Ibid.
12 'Domestic correspondence: New York letter', *JAMA*, 1885, Vol. 5, pp. 556–8.
13 J. Price, 'A system of free nursing as organized in Philadelphia', *JAMA*, 1888, Vol. 11, p. 340.
14 'The Illinois Training School for Nurses', *JAMA*, 1888, Vol. 11, pp. 705–6.
15 These were different, competing sects within US medicine. The regulars or allopaths were the mainstream medical practitioners.

16 'Address on the present status and future tendencies of the medical profession', *JAMA*, 1883, Vol. 1 (2), pp. 33–42. Quotations pp. 33 and 40.
17 'Miscellaneous', *JAMA*, 1886, Vol. 6, pp. 279–280; B. Cornick, 'The remedy for overcrowding in the medical profession', *JAMA*, 1889, Vol. 13, pp. 613–15; 'How to limit the number of medical colleges and lessen the crowded conditions of the medical profession', *JAMA*, 1888, Vol. 10, pp. 722–3; 'What is the proper mode of limiting the number of medical colleges and medical men?' *JAMA*, 1888, Vol. 10, pp. 655–6.
18 Ibid., p. 655.
19 Cornick, 'The remedy for overcrowding', p. 614.
20 'Editorial: Medical education in the United States in 1893', *JAMA*, 1896, Vol. 26, pp. 183–4.
21 'Society proceedings: General education of the physician', *JAMA*, 1891, Vol. 16, pp. 785–7.
22 'Editorial: The new nurse again', *JAMA*, 1896, Vol. 27, pp. 606–7.
23 Ibid.
24 'Minor comments: School Nurses' Society', *JAMA*, 1899, Vol. 33 (2), pp. 106–7.
25 'Book Notices: *Surgical Nursing by Bertha M. Voswinkle*', *JAMA*, 1899, Vol. 32 (14), pp. 786–7.
26 'Minor comments: The nurse's responsibility', *JAMA*, 1899, Vol. 33 (25), p. 1556.
27 'Society proceedings', *JAMA*, 1898, Vol. 31 (20), p. 1177.
28 'Society proceedings', *JAMA*, 1898, Vol. 31 (14), p. 791.
29 B. Lusk, 'Pretty and powerless: nurses in advertisements, 1930–1950', *Research in Nursing and Health*, 2000, Vol. 23, pp. 229–36.
30 'Trained female nurses for the army', *JAMA*, 1899, Vol. 32 (6), p. 329.
31 N. Senn, 'Nursing and nurses in war', *JAMA*, 1899, Vol. 32 (4), pp. 155–9.
32 Ibid.
33 'Editorial: The female nurse in the army', *JAMA*, 1899, Vol. 33 (23), pp. 1432–3.
34 Ibid.
35 Morantz, 'The "connecting link"'.
36 'Medical education in the United States', *JAMA*, 1905, Vol. 45, pp. 536–9.
37 'Medical education in the United States', *JAMA*, 1909, Vol. 53 (7), pp. 556–62.
38 'Editorial: The future of medical education in the United States', *JAMA*, 1907, Vol. 48 (19), pp. 1603–4.
39 G. H. Simmons, 'Medical education and preliminary requirements', *JAMA*, 1904, Vol. 42 (19), pp. 1205–10.
40 H. C. Putnam, 'Attendants and nursemaids', *JAMA*, 1902, Vol. 38 (21), pp. 1364–6.
41 'Current Medical Literature: The over-trained nurse', *JAMA*, 1906, Vol. 46 (9), pp. 1476.
42 'Society proceedings: The problem of efficient nursing of persons of moderate income', *JAMA*, 1909, Vol. 52 (8), p. 654.
43 Putnam, 'Attendants and nursemaids', p. 1365.
44 'Editorial: Wanted: Trained nurses for the middle classes', *JAMA*, 1909, Vol. 53 (2), p. 122.
45 'Queries and minor notes: Professions entitled to gratuitous service', *JAMA*, 1905, Vol. 45, p. 344.
46 'Minor comments: Nurses' schools and illegal practice of medicine', *JAMA*, 1906, Vol. 47 (22), p. 1835.
47 Ibid.
48 'Medical news: model rules for nurses', *JAMA*, 1911, Vol. 56 (6), p. 434.
49 J. W. Griffith, 'Don'ts for nurses' *JAMA*, 1914, Vol. 63 (25), pp. 2253–4.
50 'Medical news: Model rules for nurses', *JAMA*, 1911, Vol. 56 (6), p. 434.
51 'Book notices: Nursing Ethics, Isabel Hampton Robb', *JAMA*, 1901, Vol. 36 (17), p. 1195.
52 'Editorial: Nursing and the physician', *JAMA*, 1902, Vol. 38 (22), pp. 1443–4.

53　'The over-trained nurse, *JAMA*, 1906, Vol. 46 (14), p. 1042; 'Current Medical Literature: The over-trained nurse' *JAMA*, 1906, Vol. 46 (9), p. 1476.

54　'Current medical literature: Nurses' training schools' *JAMA*, 1901, Vol. 37 (23), p. 1560.

55　'Current medical literature: Trained nurses', *JAMA*, 1903, Vol. 41 (1), p. 56.

56　'Current medical literature: What nurses should be taught', *JAMA*, 1906, Vol. 46 (19), p. 1476.

57　'Current medical literature: Training of nurses', *JAMA*, 1906, Vol. 46 (15), p. 1139.

58　'Society proceedings: The relationship between the State Board of Regents and training schools', *JAMA*, 1910, Vol. 54 (9), p. 732.

59　'Society proceedings: American Hospital Association', *JAMA*, 1908, Vol. 51 (17), p. 1445.

60　'Preliminary education of nurses and physicians' *JAMA*, 1907, Vol. 48 (23), p. 1978.

61　M. H. McMillan, 'Correspondence: The supply of practical nurses', *JAMA*, 1919, Vol. 72 (9), p. 671.

62　M. L. Harris, 'Correspondence: Comment on McMillan's "The supply of practical nurses"', *JAMA*, 1919, Vol. 72 (9), pp. 671–2.

63　'Current comment: Press comments on the report of the Carnegie Foundation', *JAMA*, 1910, Vol. 55 (4), p. 318.

64　J. K. Mason, 'Correspondence: Need of campaign to arouse interest in trained nursing', *JAMA*, 1918, Vol. 70 (24), p. 1882; 'Editorial: The supply of nurses', *JAMA*, 1919, Vol. 72 (9), p. 657.

65　J. B. Howland, 'Obligations of hospitals and the public to training schools for nurses', *JAMA*, 1913, Vol. 61 (24), pp. 2152–4.

66　'Society Proceedings: Discussion on the nursing problem', *JAMA*, 1910, Vol. 54 (9), p. 732.

67　Ibid., p. 733.

68　E. T. Milligan, 'Letter to the editor: Need for inexpensive obstetric nurses', *JAMA*, 1913, Vol. 61 (8), p. 617.

69　R. O. Beard, 'The trained nurse of the future', *JAMA*, 1913, Vol. 61 (24), pp. 2149–52.

70　Howland, 'Obligations of hospitals'.

71　M. Ostheimer, 'The value of the social service department to the children's dispensary', *JAMA*, 1912, Vol. 59 (22), pp. 1944–6; W. H. Price, 'A year's experience with contagious disease nurses', *JAMA*, 1914, Vol. 63 (21), pp. 1811–12; 'Society Proceedings, The visiting nurse in the fight against tuberculosis', *JAMA*, 1915, Vol. 65 (25), p. 2194; 'Community nurses' *JAMA*, 1917, Vol. 68 (12), p. 892; 'The city nurse as an agent for the prevention of infant mortality', *JAMA*, 1918, Vol. 71 (25), p. 2102; 'Public health nursing', *JAMA*, 1919, Vol. 73 (7), p. 496.

72　'Medical News: More nurses for the Navy', *JAMA*, 1918, Vol. 70 (21), p. 1553; 'Medical News: Army School of Nursing', *JAMA*, 1918, Vol. 70 (24), p. 1874; 'Medical mobilization and the war', *JAMA*, 1918, Vol. 70 (25), p. 1949; 'Correspondence: The Army School of Nursing', *JAMA*, 1918, Vol. 71 (5), p. 399.

73　'Editorial: Nurses needed by the Red Cross', *JAMA*, 1918, Vol. 70 (23), p. 1768.

74　'Editorial: The supply of practical nurses', *JAMA*, 1919, Vol. 72 (4), pp. 276–7.

75　Ibid.

76　C. V. Chapin, 'Correspondence: The supply of practical nurses', *JAMA*, 1919, Vol. 72 (6), p. 442.

77　H. N. MacKechnie, 'Correspondence: The supply of practical nurses', *JAMA*, 1919, Vol. 72 (6), p. 442.

78　G. K. Dickinson, 'Correspondence: The supply of practical nurses', *JAMA*, 1919, Vol. 72 (6), p. 442.

79　A. P. Leighton, 'Correspondence: The supply of practical nurses', *JAMA*, 1919, Vol. 72 (7), p. 514.

80   P. K. Brown, 'Correspondence: The supply of practical nurses', *JAMA*, 1919, Vol. 72 (18), pp. 1316–17.

81   'Editorial: Medical education-progress of 21 years', *JAMA*, 1921, Vol. 77 (7), pp. 557–9.

82   'Editorial: Doctors of medical practice and the cost of medical care', *JAMA*, 1929, Vol. 93 (6), pp. 458–60.

83   Annual Congress on Medical Education, Medical Licensure, Public Health and Hospitals, 'Preliminary report of the committee on trained nursing to the council on medical education of the American Medical Association', *JAMA*, 1923, Vol. 80 (12), pp. 851–3; M. A. Burgess, 'The nursing shortage', *JAMA*, 1928, Vol. 90 (12), pp. 898–900.

84   'Correspondence: T.F.B. Supply of nurses', *JAMA*, 1920, Vol. 75 (23), p. 1585.

85   'Cooperation of medical and nursing organisations for the solution of nursing problems', *JAMA*, 1920, Vol. 74 (22), p. 1537.

86   'Medical news: Drive for student nurses', *JAMA*, 1921, Vol. 76 (9), p. 600.

87   'Minutes of House of Delegates: Address of President-elect, William Allen Pusey', *JAMA*, 1924. Vol. 82 (24), pp. 1960–4.

88   Ibid.

89   'Editorial: Trained nurses', *JAMA*, 1926, Vol. 86 (24), p. 1841.

90   'Correspondence: Nurses records and home nursing', *JAMA*, 1927, Vol. 89 (7), p. 542.

91   G. C. Stimpson, 'Correspondence: Nurses and nursing', *JAMA*, 1927, Vol. 89 (13), pp. 1078–9.

92   J. D. Robertson, 'Social medicine and medical economics: Home and public health nurses and their training', *JAMA*, 1920, Vol. 74 (7), pp. 481–3.

93   W. J. Mayo, 'Observations on South America' *JAMA*, 1920, Vol. 75 (5), pp. 311–15.

94   'Editorial: The nursing problem', *JAMA*, 1920, Vol. 75 (5), p. 324.

95   'Medical news: High cost of nursing', *JAMA*, 1926, Vol. 86 (16), pp. 1223–4.

96   R. O. Beard, 'Minority report of committee on trained nursing', *JAMA*, 1923, Vol. 80 (12), pp. 852–3.

97   Ibid.

98   'Minutes of House of Delegates: Report of special reference committee on nursing education', *JAMA*, 1927, Vol. 88 (22), p. 1732.

99   'Report of committee on nurses and nursing education', *JAMA*, 1927, Vol. 88 (15), pp. 1175–80.

100 'Proceedings of the Washington Session: Address of the speaker, Dr. F. C. Warnshuis', *JAMA*, 1927, Vol. 88 (21), pp. 1642–3.

101 'Medical News: New York Report of Committee on Nursing', *JAMA*, 1928, Vol. 91 (2), pp. 103–4.

102 'Medical News: Michigan, Committee's Report on Nursing Service', *JAMA*, 1928, Vol. 91 (17), p. 1296.

103 'Book notices: Gladys Sellew, "Pediatric nursing including the nursing care of the well infant and child".' *JAMA*, 1927, Vol. 88 (5), p. 346.

104 'Book notices: M. Adelaide Nutting, A sound economic basis for schools of nursing and other addresses', *JAMA*, 1927, Vol. 88 (15), p. 1202.

105 W. Darrach, 'Reports of officers: Report of the Committee on the Grading of Nursing Schools', *JAMA*, 1928, Vol. 90 (18), p. 1477; M.A. Burgess, 'The nursing shortage', *JAMA*, 1928, Vol. 90 (12), pp. 898–900.

106 'Editorial: The cost of medical care', *JAMA*, 1930, Vol. 94 (2), p. 106.

107 M. M. Davis, 'Doctors' bills and peoples billions', *JAMA*, 1930, Vol. 94 (13), pp. 1014–17.

108 'Address of President M. L. Harris', *JAMA*, 1930, Vol. 94, (26), pp. 2070–2.

109 W. G. Morgan, 'President's address. The medical profession and the paternalistic tendencies of the times', *JAMA*, 1930, Vol. 94 (26), pp. 2035–42.

110 'Editorial: The Committee on the Costs of Medical Care', *JAMA*, 1932, Vol. 99 (23), pp. 1950–2; 'Final report of the Committee on the Costs of Medical Care', *JAMA*, 1932, Vol. 99 (23), pp. 1953–8.
111 'Book Notices: Nursing schools today and tomorrow', *JAMA*, 1935, Vol. 104 (2), p. 142.
112 'Editorial: Nursing Education', *JAMA*, 1934, Vol. 103 (14), p. 1070.

7 Race, identity and the nursing profession in South Africa, c. 1850–1958

Helen Sweet and Anne Digby[1]

You may already have heard of the threatened Nurses Strike here at Sulenkama. It "broke" on 3rd June [1949] . . . That morning every probationer nurse was sitting by the roadside with her cases packed at 6 a.m., waiting for the bus, and leaving a fairly full hospital quite unattended. Had they carried out their intention we would have had no alternative but to stop admitting patients and gradually to empty the hospital . . . Prompt action and the guiding action of God saved the situation.[2]

Historically, strike action by nurses has been, and still is, quite unusual. But moments of crisis and confrontation expose issues otherwise obscured by such factors as the ordered hierarchy of a hospital, the distribution of power between White and Black, or inequalities between men and women. In the case of the Sulenkama mission hospital, to be discussed in our case study, the causes of disaffection among these young, Black nurses revealed a complex layering of issues, so that an unpublicized event at an obscure mission hospital serves as a lens to clarify some of the stresses within the South African nursing profession. The first section of this chapter places South African nurses in historical perspective, highlighting the growth of qualified Black nurses, and the way in which mission hospitals played an important early role in their training; the second section provides an analytical narrative of the incidents at Sulenkama and the final section brings these two perspectives together in reflecting on professional development within a context of transcultural nursing studies.

THE DEVELOPMENT OF A DIVIDED NURSING PROFESSION

Nursing in South Africa developed in a fragmented way. Provision of domestic nursing care for Dutch and British families ranged from approved Dutch midwives to the untrained female slaves and family members of settlers and lay care providers, all of whom practised rudimentary home nursing and used folk remedies, patent medicines and herbal treatments.[3] African health care was provided by an equally diverse range of indigenous practitioners, with nursing of the sick shared between family members and the 'wise women' of the community, who might also practise as traditional childbirth attendants.[4] Institutional nursing developed gradually. By the nineteenth century, military hospitals employed their own (predominantly white, male) nurses whereas emerging civilian hospitals used a mixture of Black and Cape coloured women as assistant nurses for more menial duties.[5] In King William's Town in the 1860s, Dr Fitzgerald, the Superintendent of a pioneering hospital, began training African women to nurse Black hospital patients. Not until the late nineteenth century did the first trained White nurses arrive from Europe,[6] a move that reflected reforms in nursing taking place there that were opening up possibilities for nursing as a career for educated women.[7] Part of the underlying proselytizing purpose of this movement was to use nurses to spread ideals of nursing and sanitary reform throughout the Empire.[8] These changes also promoted a system of hierarchical order and discipline based on differentials in class, gender, and where appropriate, also in racial difference.

Religious sisterhoods had an important role in these early institutions. The Albany Hospital in Grahamstown, which was established in 1850, was staffed by Roman Catholic nuns from the Order of the Assumption. In 1871 Anglican Sisters provided nursing care for the New Somerset Hospital in Cape Town and its trained nurses then replaced or supervised untrained staff.[9] In Bloemfontein, the Anglican sisterhood of St Michael began to provide nursing care for those working in the diamond fields at Kimberley. Sister Henrietta Stockdale emerged from this religious order as the pioneer in establishing nurse education and registration.[10] Shula Marks has interpreted Henrietta Stockdale's real and mythic significance in South African nursing history as being much like that of Florence Nightingale in British nursing history.[11] Charlotte Searle has argued that the particularities of nurse training in South Africa resulted from insufficient numbers of medical practitioners in rural areas, which often required the nurse 'to step into the breach and take on the total health care of the patient'.[12]

Particularly significant in the later training of Black nurses were the mission hospitals that were built from the end of the nineteenth century, the first of these was Victoria Hospital, Lovedale, built in 1898.[13] It trained the first Black registered nurse, Cecilia Makiwane, in 1908, and for many years was the most important centre for educating African nurses. Thereafter, as Mashaba comments, 'Training of professional nurses progressed slowly – mainly because of lack of suitably qualified candidates. Most of the Black girls who were suitably educated were being recruited into the teaching profession.'[14] Nurse-probationers were exposed to strict discipline and there appears to have been little understanding by White nursing supervisors of the cross-cultural problems they faced. Smaller mission hospitals were strongly motivated to train African nurses – partly for functional reasons (to provide staff for hospitals situated in remote areas) and partly for idealistic ones (as a means of uplifting and educating Africans). But these institutions found it difficult to obtain probationers of a sufficiently high educational standard to pass nursing examinations that had to be taken in English or Afrikaans, regardless of the first language of the nurse. They also faced problems in retaining staff because they could not offer the attractively wide range of experience of larger, well-equipped, urban hospitals.

Although a general shortage of nurses was one important motivating factor in developing training schemes in South Africa, some of the specific impetus for training Black nurses originated from racist attitudes towards patient care. This was epitomized by a comment in the *Transvaal Medical Journal* in 1912 that: 'There can be no doubt that for European women to wait on natives is highly undesirable, and for young nurses to be in charge of, or to nurse in, male Kaffir wards is nothing short of criminal.'[15] This was a contested view, as subsequent correspondence indicated. A Johannesburg doctor condemned this argument as racist and described how White nurses had successfully nursed Black patients at his hospital for the last 20 years without 'one instance of disrespect or of improper conduct of a native patient towards a nurse'.[16]

It was not until the mid-1920s that a more concerted interest was taken in the need for nurse training by the government. In 1925, a hospital inquiry appointed by the Minister of Health recommended 'the training of Native nurses and midwives with the same standard as that of Europeans'.[17] In 1928, the Loram Committee also 'reported in favour of full training' for nursing and medicine, recommending that village 'nursing stations' should be staffed with an African health assistant and an African nurse-midwife with cooperation from mission hospitals.[18] However, by the early 1930s a greater note of urgency can be detected in discussions on the need to recruit and train African nurses to work in public health and children's health and welfare (Figure 7.1).

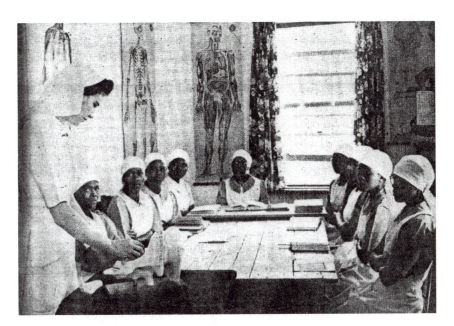

Figure 7.1   Photograph showing a mission hospital classroom *c*. 1930s. From a missionary annual newsletter of the Jane Furse Hospital.

Table 7.1 Employment opportunities for 'non-European' nurses (i.e. non-White) in municipalities

	'Native'	'Coloured'
Fully qualified general nurses	11	2
Fully qualified midwives	7	3
Hospital certificate only	2	1

An important conference was held at Bloemfontein in June 1932 expressly to consider the medical services provided for, and training and employment of, 'non-Europeans'; the possibility of accepting a two-tiered system of nursing training for Whites and Blacks was hotly debated.[19] A pre-conference survey of sixty-seven hospitals (of which sixty-one had replied) provided the following data relating to 'non-European' nurses in training: fifty-seven students were studying for the General Nursing Certificate of the South African Medical Council, twenty-five students for its Midwifery Certificate and 125 students for the Hospital Certificate awarded by individual (usually mission) hospitals. Figures for the employment of non-European nurses showed that posts were not easily found and that municipalities were heavily biased against any hospital certificate that was not endorsed by the full (State Registered) nursing certificate. Yet in many areas it was not possible to obtain this because the local hospitals were small, poorly equipped missions only recognized as suitable for preparation for a Hospital Certificate. Out of 251 municipalities circularized, 183 replied, disclosing that only twenty-two of them employed non-European nurses. Of these nurses, thirty-four were described as 'native' and six as 'coloured'. This was further broken down in the interesting but incomplete analysis shown in Table 7.1. In addition to municipal employment, a few African nurses were also employed by child welfare societies.

Interestingly, following the Bloemfontein Conference, a letter was sent to the Chairman of the Board of Johannesburg General Hospital reaffirming the conference's resolutions in favour of training native nurses 'for the ordinary certificates of the Union Medical Council' and drawing the Board's attention to recent high pass rates in general nursing and midwifery examinations at Lovedale, the American Board Hospital in Durban and the Bridgeman Memorial Hospital, Johannesburg.[20] The letter pointed to the desirability of employing fully trained nurses wherever possible and urged the Board to begin training, 'non-European nurses for the General Nursing Certificate of the Medical Council'. A central point of the correspondence was also to answer the Board's claim regarding, 'grave complaints that native nurses refuse to accept responsibility.' In defence of the nurses, the letter suggested that these are 'probationers who are not qualified educationally to proceed to the full training . . . *In any case, the sense of responsibility must be less where the training is less thorough*' (emphasis in original). This comment is especially relevant to later events at the hospital at Sulenkama to which we now turn.

NESSIE KNIGHT HOSPITAL, SULENKAMA

The institution at Sulenkama was one among many mission hospitals, whose individual character and ethos varied. The nurses' strike at the Nessie Knight Hospital at Sulenkama has not yet achieved historical visibility, but archival material located within the National Library of Scotland enables the nursing historian to construct a very detailed picture of one set of encounters between Black nurses and their White superiors in South Africa.

A mission hospital such as Sulenkama might not be expected to occupy a prominent place in any pathology of institutions. For was such an establishment not filled with 'Godly people', strongly motivated to do good and to show by the force of their life of service, and even more by their power of healing, that the Gospel was truth? Were not the doctors and nurses following in the footsteps of Christ – the very first medical missionary? Yet the small size of such medical missions meant that any personality conflict among the staff tended to fester. The problem of attracting sufficient staff to serve in remote locations added to the stress caused by tiredness and inadequate rest periods or furloughs. In addition, ambitious plans to expand facilities to meet a buoyant demand for medical treatment should have been constrained, given the enduring financial problems, but the imperatives of medical evangelism meant that these were seldom heeded, and stress was compounded through continued anxieties as to whether commitments could be sustained. In these conflicted circumstances it was not unusual to find that, whereas the mission achieved a great deal of good for many disadvantaged patients, it provided a tense and unhappy working environment for its staff.

Sulenkama was a clear exemplar of this functional duality. Robert Paterson, a recent medical graduate from Glasgow University, then twenty-five years old, had gone out to Sulenkama in 1927 and three years later a twelve-bed hospital was opened. Fifteen years later it had 100 beds and the 182 in-patients of its first year soon grew to 300.[21] Outward appearances suggested that this was a success story, and Michael Gelfand's brief, but positive, published description reflects this public facade.[22] Yet private correspondence from, and about, the hospital gives a strikingly different impression, and one that makes the action of its nurses more understandable.[23] A secretary dismissed by Dr Paterson for 'disloyalty' in 1948, the year before the nurses' strike, wrote to the mission authorities in Scotland:

> I cannot say I am sorry to leave Sulenkama for there are certain elements in its make-up which do not make for happiness . . . If the Church of Scotland feels that the amount of unhappiness experienced here is normal on the Mission Field, and must be – because of the type of life – and that it has no repercussion on the evangelistic side in the mind and heart of the African – then people will go and come and come and go here.[24]

However, the unwholesome crucible of institutional life also provided huge stresses for Sulenkama's Medical Superintendent, who suffered increasingly serious mental and physical health problems. Seven years later this resulted in the mission society dismissing him.[25]

Institutions such as hospitals also facilitated political organization by the discontented. Shula Marks has analysed an early incident in 1921 involving Black nurses at a mine hospital on the Rand that highlighted the issue of expectations in relation to working and living conditions. Among the nurses' grievances was the fact that they were not satisfied with the quality of their food, the restrictive regulations on their laundry or their limited time off. As at Sulenkama, Black nurses saw themselves as an educated elite and were not prepared to acquiesce in the kind of working conditions tolerated by the male Black nursing orderlies who had been recruited from ordinary migrant mine labour. Significantly, many of these female nurses had been educated at the premier training institution of Lovedale. Their intractability took mine officials by surprise. Similar cases of indiscipline and insubordination occurred through the 1920s and into the 1930s and led to the imposition of much stricter discipline.[26]

By the 1940s, official anxiety was expressed about this kind of African unrest. In 1943, several disturbances occurred in institutions, including one among patients and employees at Fort Beaufort Hospital, the asylum for Black patients in the Eastern Cape, where police and army volunteers had to be called in to restore order.[27] The Second World War had been fought for a better world and disaffection followed disappointed hopes; young people – both students and nurses – emerged in radical roles. Marks has referred to the 'very widespread disaffection' in African high schools during the 1940s and has analysed events in 1947 at a mission boarding school, Adams High School, in Natal, where student boycotts first caused an unpopular head teacher to resign and then resulted in 175 students being sent home.[28] In the following year, the electoral success of the National Party led to the implementation of apartheid policies that in turn generated a new and more radical political mood among Africans. This frame of mind meant that concrete grievances could soon provide the pretext for radical action, and the enclosed world of institutions provided a theatre for confrontation. Over a longer time period, John Hyslop has also noted the prevalence of Black unrest in a range of institutions, and has pointed out that food and domestic labour were frequent trigger-points of disturbances;[29] the latter was an important issue at Sulenkama.

Events at educational and medical institutions of missions in the eastern Cape to the south of Sulenkama provide a regional context for the strike threatened by nurses at Sulenkama. At St Matthew's College, Keiskammahoek, there was arson, riot and resistance in 1945, and in 1949 the matron noted that there was 'a girl's war' among teacher trainees at St Matthews, who actively flouted gender expectations by indulging in violence and vandalism.[30] In a penetrating study of Lovedale, Anne Mager found a similar pattern of girls at first supporting more active boys during the riots of August 1946 that closed the school, and then a second and more violent disturbance in 1949 when the girls showed more active defiance. At Lovedale's Victoria Hospital, a probationer nurse challenged her superior and was dismissed. This action provoked a strike that led to the dismissal of all student nurses because they would not recognize the authority of the hospital hierarchy, and resulted in a prolonged closure of the hospital.[31] Clearly, at these two institutions girls became increasingly assertive during the 1940s.

Lovedale (including the Victoria Hospital there) was the flagship among mission institutions run by the Church of Scotland. It was the first of a small chain of medical missions that ran from the eastern Cape to the northern frontier of South Africa, with Sulenkama being the next hospital in line north of Lovedale (Figure 7.2). Dr Paterson, the first Sulenkama Medical Superintendent, had visited Victoria Hospital on the way to his first post and cordial relationships continued between the two institutions. That a strike in the middle of May at Lovedale was followed by one in early June at Sulenkama was hardly coincidental. This was part of a more general heightening of political consciousness among young African women in nursing. In 1947 there had been a twelve-day nurses' strike at the Clinic in Alexandra township in Johannesburg, and at Baragwanath Hospital in the same city in July 1949. A strike was narrowly averted in a confrontation between senior White and junior non-European staff, which occurred only a month after the strike at Sulenkama.[32]

Dr Paterson blamed wider societal developments for the threat of strike action by Black nurses at Sulenkama. 'That there is a great deal of unrest among the Bantu just now, is part at any rate of the kernel of the affair.'[33] He was undoubtedly correct in this diagnosis but his recourse to external influences as a key cause

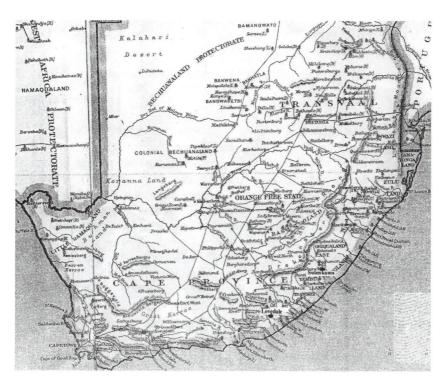

Figure 7.2   Map of South Africa *c.* 1911 showing mission stations and Lovedale and Sulenkama mission hospitals. From the London Geographical Institute, published by Longmans, Green and Co. (London).

of the strike was also psychologically revealing. Intensely proud of the growing hospital with its 'lovely new Nurses Home' he was reluctant to analyse difficulties nearer home. Although devising structural reforms to solve an institutional problem, he looked primarily to personal influence to effect social control. 'My wife has always had a wonderful influence with our African nurses for the simple reason that she does genuinely love them, and they know it. So when she returns [from sick leave] I am hoping we will have no further trouble.'[34]

From the young African nurses, whose frustrations had precipitated the strike, different issues emerged in a letter delivered to the superintendent's house thirty-six hours before the strike:

> Sir,
>
> The complaints run as follows: (1) We are working very hard, e.g. (the domestic work) polishing, laundry, and kitchens etc. (2) Preparatories [i.e. Probationers] not wanted by the Sister in Charge and beginners and juniors are not allowed to take temperatures, giving of medicines, nor treatments. How will they be perfect? As we believe that practice makes perfect. (3) We would like to know the difference between a nurse and a worker in your hospital, e.g. working with the workers in the field. (4) Vulgar language used on nurses, called pigs, brass monkeys, and Africans with little education. ALL THIS WE ASK IN LOVE. We would like all these to be abolished. Doctor we can be pleased if you can answer us tomorrow.
>
> We remain,
>
> Your Nurses.[35]

The dominant theme here was one of contested identity in that the nurses desired a legitimacy that they thought was being denied to them. This aspiration was shaped by an awareness of their perceived identity, because African girls recruited into nurse training programmes were part of an educated elite that was working towards a privileged professional position. As such, they tended to value knowledge from books as superior to inferior practical work.[36] But at Sulenkama they were confronted by a situation that subverted their ambitions – they had to do manual work, not just within the hospital but, even more humiliatingly, in the fields outside it. At the same time they were given restricted opportunities to practise the nursing care that would have advanced their training, instead being given demeaning, routine hospital tasks. Terms of abuse shamed and dishonoured them but also cemented their subordinate identity into an inferior position in a racial hierarchy. These cumulated mortifications forged a political consciousness that informed their radical decision to strike.

The response to complaints by the nurses suggests the unequal distribution of power in a mission hospital. Dr Paterson undertook to discontinue any domestic work that student nurses were doing in the houses of their White superiors. And, although justifying work in the fields on the grounds that it had been started for the health of the nurses, agreed that it should be discontinued. But he made clear that the necessity for nurses to do domestic work in the hospital was non-negotiable, although making an attempt to sweeten the pill. 'Once the *essential* domestic work of the wards is *done*, then we are quite willing that Preparatories be allowed into the wards to do this work, and at the same time by keeping their eyes and ears open they can also be learning the routine work of the wards.'[37] (emphasis as in the original). Given that there were few trained White staff to supervise Black nurses, much was made of their earlier inefficiencies and lack of attention as a justification for their marginal position on the wards. After talking to the senior White nursing officer, Sister Collins, Dr Patterson recorded that:

> Temperatures *must* be accurate, and we have found a good deal of inaccuracy in the past. . .Medicines *must* be accurately measured and carefully given. Sister has found pills and tablets lying on the beds and on the patients' lockers, i.e. the nurse has just handed them out but has not waited to make sure that the patient takes them. Treatments: We have found many instances of burns from hot water bottles, of bedsores developing through careless lack of attention.[38]

Despite these allegations Dr Paterson, persuaded Sister Collins that in future more nursing practice by juniors should be offered, providing only that senior trainee nurses supervised the taking of temperatures and the administration of medicines and treatments.

Racially differentiated practices were easier to redress than racist attitudes. In consultation with his White colleagues, Paterson admitted that 'the African Nurses could be and often were irritating and that . . . I had frequently lost my temper with them, but . . . I have never used any of the terms complained of by the Nurses . . . I have long since learned that the Bantu are peculiarly sensitive to being called names.' It is at least a possibility that the nurses had misheard the abusive terms they complained about, since 'brass monkeys' makes little sense in this context. Whatever the reality here, the doctor considered that it would be counterproductive to find out which White member of staff had been impolite but assured his aggrieved Black nurses that henceforward no one would employ these abusive terms.

Attempting to persuade the Black nurses to call off their threatened strike, Dr Paterson used a variety of approaches that fortuitously provide us with a clear insight into what had deteriorated into a repressive regime concealed by a rhetorical facade of affectionate concern. Paterson was the main speaker at a meeting on the evening of 3 June, although he invited Dr Currie, as well as Sister Collins, to reinforce his message. Dr Paterson opened the meeting with customary forms of mission discourse. 'What I have to say I say to you in love. In true love for your own good.' This was addressed to what he admitted were silent, sullen and resentful nurses. Initially he adopted tactics of divide and rule by pointing out that 'there are hotheads and agitators among you who have stirred up this trouble, and some of you are allowing yourselves to be led astray.' Then came a detailed exposition of the legal position of the nurses, their signed agreement to do nursing, agricultural and domestic work, and the need for a month's notice if they wished to leave. The doctor next adopted an overtly threatening tone by admonishing his listeners that, if they continued to follow their current line of conduct, 'you would find that you couldn't get into any other decent hospital, as we would send a list with all your names to every [other] hospital'. Also, that if the nurses left without the obligatory month's notice 'there is a law in this country whereby you can be arrested and prosecuted.' Not content with secular coercion, Paterson reminded them of divine retribution, 'Your earthly judge would have no mercy on nurses who deserted their patients. I leave it to yourselves to imagine what your heavenly judge would think about it.' Having spent most of the meeting being tough he finally reverted to his initial, tender mode. 'I am still your friend. Help me to continue to be your friend. Nessie [his wife] – always loved the nurses (always tried to save them from dismissal.) If you do anything foolish it will break her heart. Think what you are doing!'[39]

After discovering the following morning that his arguments had been ineffective and that the nurses were at the bus stop about to leave, Paterson turned to external means of persuasion or coercion. Aware that the nurses came from a socially conservative African background he turned first to Chief Isaac Matiwane. He and the hospital's African minister, Reverend N'tuli, were asked to speak to the girls, and the local teacher, Felix Jubase, hastened to join them. Not having absolute confidence in the utility of his first line of attack, Dr Paterson then had recourse to the world of White officialdom. He drove to Qumbu to fetch the magistrate and the public prosecutor. On the drive back, he was reassured to learn that he had been technically correct in warning the nurses that they were liable to arrest and imprisonment under the Masters and Servants Act that attached criminal liability to a civil contract. (Strikes by nurses were not made illegal in South Africa until 1978.) Meanwhile, during his absence, the Chief had been talking to the nurses. The magistrate explained to the nurses their legal liabilities and then the Chief and teacher talked with the nurses by themselves. This was apparently fruitful because, on their return to the main meeting, the nurses agreed to go on with the work of the hospital.

A gendered reading of these events would indicate its patriarchal character, because ultimate authority was very much vested in men, whether African or European. However, white women also played vital – if secondary – roles, whether this was the day-to-day ordering of the nurses' day on the wards by Sister Collins or the domestic oversight of the hospital by Nessie Paterson. Throughout this difficult period, Dr Paterson attempted to make the young nurses aware of the absent Nessie Paterson's 'maternal' care:

> *Inkosikazi* – your mother in Sulenkama . . . When *Inkosikazi* comes back you can speak to her as to a mother. Meanwhile you can speak to me as your father. Your own fathers and mothers would have been greatly upset if we had had to write and tell them that the hospital was closed because of what you were going to do.[40]

Paterson showed only limited political acumen in aligning the socially conservative regime of the mission hospital to that of the girls' own families, because recent social change was developing generational differences in African society between youthful activists and more conservative parents. These young Black nurses were caught between rival pressures, as can be seen in their statement of grievances in which a tension is evident between an accustomed language of deference and a newly discovered, assertive self-confidence.

Dr Paterson admitted that problems in running Sulenkama Hospital were sometimes 'quite unbearable'.[41] Situated in the Transkei, the institution was geographically remote and, like other South African mission hospitals, this isolation exacerbated recruitment problems. Perpetual shortage of staff helps explain its routines of 'divine drudgery' and thus why nurse training was, at best, geared towards domestic labour and, at worst, undercut by it. There was an obvious parallel in the causes of the strikes by nurses at both Sulenkama and Lovedale over the deployment of African probationers as domestic workers. A male student at Fort Hare referred to the 'sheer exploitation' of the Lovedale student nurses.[42] And in 1949, Robert Sobukwe, a prominent Black member of the African National Congress (ANC) Youth League (then spearheading the radicalization of the ANC) placed the actions of the nurses at Lovedale in the context of a developing power struggle between Black and White in apartheid South Africa:

> The trouble at the Hospital . . . should be viewed as part of a broad struggle and not as an isolated incident . . . We must fight for freedom – for the right to call our souls our own. And we must pay the price. The nurses have paid the price.[43]

The South African Nursing Council Board, which was composed only of White members, gave an alternative verdict on the Lovedale strike. Despite acknowledging that the grievances of the African nurses were largely substantiated, it condemned the strike action as 'a gross breach of the ethical standards of the nursing profession'. That strikes by nurses were regarded as unprofessional was a perception aligned with more general social attitudes expressing shock and displeasure. For example, an earlier stoppage by Black probationer nurses at Sir Henry Elliot Hospital, Umtata, in 1941 was similarly reported in the *Territorial News* as 'unheard of' and 'besmirching' the 'great profession [of nursing]'. Yet strikes by nurses were not isolated incidents in South Africa. White nurses had threatened strike action in 1924 at Addington,[44] and three years later White nurses had actually struck at Victoria Hospital, Mafikeng, in a well-publicized protest against having to work with a Black practitioner, Dr Molema. Unrest continued in hospitals. There was another strike by nurses at Victoria Hospital, Lovedale, in 1958, when 100 out of 140 Black nurses held a mass sit-down strike after a staff nurse colleague was expelled; this incident resulted in the expulsion of nurses and the suspension of nurse training.

This last incident has been located firmly within a transcultural context by Mashaba who suggested that this – and many other internal conflicts that were more successfully contained – 'stemmed from a lack of communication and con-sultation at a local level' . . . because 'white nurses who held matrons' positions in some hospitals had no understanding of the problems of some of the Black nurses.'[45] The problem of cross-cultural understanding had also been highlighted in connection with the earlier Mafikeng strike. Dr C. Louis Leipoldt, the liberal editor of the *South African Medical Journal*, stated that 'we know that the col-our bar is only one of many retrogressive methods that may be used in panic by those who are doubtful of their own ability and power'.[46] In important respects, Mafikeng was a mirror image of the Sulenkama and Lovedale strikes. Within an increasingly segregated society, the Mafikeng protest by white nurses was directed towards the threat of an established racial hierarchy being inverted. In Sulenkama and Lovedale the problem lay in the unequal relationships being strictly enforced in the hospitals when racial order was being challenged within a wider society.

SIGNIFICANT ISSUES

Writing in 2002, the editor of *Nursing Update* and *Curationis* stated (emphasis added):

> The challenge for [South African] nurses, therefore, is to ensure that the stand-ard and quality of care at public health institutions is not undermined, *either by themselves or by the policies of the government of the day*. They have to hold the government accountable to their undertakings. The second challenge is for nursing academics and historians to begin seriously to look at writing and recording the work of all those nurses who have contributed towards the formation and development of the nursing profession. *The history of nursing in this country has to reflect all its people and not just a segment of them.*[47]

This short chapter has accepted this challenge to write inclusive nursing history by taking a significant episode, the nurses attempted strike at Sulenkama in 1949, and using it to illustrate some of the issues of status and identity encountered in the early development of a South African nursing profession that included only 800 Black nurses at that time.

Shula Marks has perceptively pointed out that Black South African nurses were all too often 'the most visible scapegoat' for intolerable strains in hospitals.[48] A condemnatory attitude towards nurses taking strike action has certainly not been confined to South Africa and it would appear to be universal even today, both as a knee-jerk media response and as a more considered reaction from within the profession to what is perceived to be a tarnishing of the (stereotypical) image of nursing as a vocational calling with self-sacrifice and philanthropy at its founda-tion. A description of the 1937 march of masked nurses in London who hid their identities 'for fear of victimization'[49] but protested against low pay, staff shortages and long hours of work, epitomizes this unacceptable face of nursing.

In whatever country it was situated, nursing during the first half of the twen-tieth century encountered considerable problems. The varied socio-economic backgrounds of nurses were lived out within an extremely hierarchical structure in which nurses were engaged in a struggle for professional autonomy. Their professional struggle was confronted by a dominant medical profession and inter-professional rivalries among nursing sub-professions. However, the racial and in-stitutional tensions, which appear to have sparked off the nursing strikes explored in this chapter, give an added transcultural dimension to these issues.

Early moves from the medical and nursing professions in South Africa to intro-duce training for African doctors and nurses, as well as lower grades of 'medical assistants' and 'nursing aids', usually restricted the argument to the premise that these trained personnel would provide health care primarily, or entirely, for the Black community in the African 'locations' and rural areas. Part of the rationale was also to try to displace indigenous healers.[50] Racism and racial segregation thus existed within the field of health care before the election of the National Party to government in 1948. Apartheid laws legitimized inequality and segregation as government policy further fragmented healthcare provision and formally divided professional representative bodies.[51]

Nurses in South Africa belonged to a divided profession. The South African Trained Nurses Association withheld full membership of the Association from trained Black or Coloured nurses, who were permitted only affiliate membership through the Bantu Trained Nurses Association. Analysing this 'divided sister-hood', Marks saw 'contradictions between the "common-sense" racism and the universalist ideology of the nursing profession.' Although fighting for fair pay and conditions and due professional respect for non-European nurses, the White leadership of the nursing profession nevertheless defended the higher status of European nurses and jealously guarded its standards against the introduction of a lesser qualification for Black and Coloured nurses.[52] Non-European nurses were placed within a spiral of inequalities because, even when fully qualified, they were forced to accept a considerable differentiation in salary compared with their White colleagues, and this situation was compounded by considerably less op-portunity to acquire specialist experience and hence gain promotion. For young probationer nurses at the Nessie Knight Hospital, Sulenkama, contemporary un-rest among young Africans during the 1940s probably tipped the balance towards activism. Already struggling to cope with the very alien tight discipline and con-trol of a mission hospital, they knew that a hospital nursing certificate was the first step in their professional careers, yet this was impeded by the non-nursing duties imposed upon them.

More generally, South African nurse leaders appear to have tried to respond to their inequitable situation through adopting diplomacy and negotiation rather than through confrontation and industrial action. For example, Alina Lekgetha, leader of the local branch of the Bantu Nurses Association at McCord Hospital in the 1940s and first Chairman of the Advisory Committee for black nurses of the South African Nursing Association (SANA), commented forcefully in 1960, 'you are not a politician you work in a political milieu'.[53] She was 'against strikes (the patient comes first) and the path of angry or emotional outbursts' yet fought for better conditions for Black nurses. Lekgetha saw 'nursing as a mission for the healing of ignorance about health, and as a mission for uplifting her people, for nursing was seen as part of the social development of the people she served'. Nevertheless she openly opposed the divisive Nursing Act (Act No. 69 of 1957) that introduced separate, racially constructed nursing registers, commenting about the meeting ' "they weren't kind to us" and we were in fact asked "in a baasskap fashion" why the Black nurse should be consulted.'[54] However, she expressed the belief that, in forcing the Black nurses to form their own branches, they were also (unintentionally) compelled to acquire and hone the professional skills and knowledge needed to run a professional association that might have been denied to them in the bigger, White-dominated body of the SANA.

In the multiracial society of South Africa, a transcultural dimension informs a large number of issues in the history of nursing and, within the brief confines of this chapter, we have highlighted only selected aspects of the problems involved when nurses move from one culture to another.[55] We have placed the spotlight on tensions between Black and White, yet we acknowledge that there are other divisive issues. One question raised as early as 1932 in relation to the education of African nurses, was whether training in a hospital would mean that Black nurses would not 'willingly go back and work among their own people'.[56] This aspect of nursing received some confirmation in a statement by a Black nurse almost forty years later – 'we do not associate ourselves with the people'.[57] Their acculturation in a Western-style hospital had thus served to distance some Black nurses from the majority of their own people and contributed towards the development of a Black bourgeois elite who lived, intermarried and socialized with similar professionals. But there were many counter-examples, particularly among community nurses, whose commitment to overcoming public health problems in disadvantaged townships was – and is – exemplary. The legacy of the pioneer of Black nursing, Cecilia Makiwane, is a powerful inspiration, not least because her example is perpetuated in the Cecilia Makiwane Nursing Awards. President Thabo Mbeki has recently acknowledged that Makiwane is 'a pioneer and a transformer [whose] qualities speak to many of us in this time of change.'[58]

NOTES

1   We would like to thank Shula Marks for her very helpful comments. We also appreciate the support of the Wellcome Trust in funding this research.
2   National Library of Scotland (henceforth NLS) 1949, accession 7548, D86–8 Sulenkama Hospital, letter to Dr A. Kerr, Secretary of South African Mission Council from Dr R. L. Paterson, Medical Superintendent of Nessie Knight Hospital Sulenkama, 20 June 1949.
3   H. C. J. Van Rensburg, E. Pretorius and A. Fourie, *Health Care in South Africa. Structure and Dynamics,* Pretoria: Academia, 1992, pp. 38–40, give the earliest approved practising midwife's arrival at the Cape as early as 1675.
4   Ibid., pp. 50–1.
5   H. Deacon, 'Outside the profession: nursing staff on Robben Island, 1846–1910', in J. Robinson, A. M. Rafferty and R. Elkan (eds), *Nursing History and the Politics of Welfare,* London: Routledge, 1997. Deacon warns against too much generalization by demonstrating that Robben Island did not always conform to the general trend.

6   Ibid., pp. 45–6, records that 'two professionally trained nurses from England assumed duty at the Provincial Hospital in Port Elizabeth in 1874'.
7   B. Abel-Smith, *A History of the Nursing Profession,* London: Heinemann, 1960, p. 17, describes this reform as involving 'changes in recruitment, changes in organisation, and even changes in the system of hospital administration'.
8   M. Baly, *Nursing and Social Change,* London: Heinemann, 1980, pp. 74–5.
9   S. Marks, *Divided Sisterhood: Race, Class and Gender in the South African Nursing Profession,* Basingstoke: St Martin's Press, 1994, p. 20. Sister Helen Bowden from University College Hospital, London, was appointed matron and strongly upheld the Nightingale nursing ethos.
10 Training began at Kimberley from 1877, and South Africa was the first country to introduce state registration for nurses in 1891 under the Medical Act No. 34 (1891) passed by the Cape colonial government and reinforced by a similar act in Natal in 1899. This legislation did not refer to race so that, at least in theory, Black women were able to train and register as nurses although none were trained at Kimberley during this period.
11 Marks, *Divided Sisterhood,* p. 16.
12 C. Searle, 'Truths that endure – faith, greatness of spirit, vision, courage and moral values', paper delivered at Potchefstroom University for Christian Higher Education, Henrietta Stockdale Memorial Lecture, 1987.
13 Elim Hospital followed one year later, in 1899, and a second wave of mission hospitals followed in the 1920s and 1930s, such as Jane Furse Hospital in the Transvaal in 1921, St. Matthew's Hospital, Keiskammahoek, in 1923, Batlaharos near Kuruman in 1932, and Mount Coke, E. Cape, in 1933.
14 T. G. Mashaba, *Rising to the Challenge of Change. A History of Black Nursing in South Africa,* Kenwyn: Juta, 1995, pp. 13–14.
15 Editorial, 'Female European nurses in male native wards', *Transvaal Medical Journal,* 1912, Vol. VIII, pp. 93–4.
16 Correspondence: H. T. Mursell, 'Female European nurses in male native wards', *Transvaal Medical Journal,* 1912, Vol. VIII, pp. 145–6.
17 'Report of Committee of Inquiry re Hospitals', *South African Medical Record,* 1925, Vol. XXIII, 12, pp. 262–4, refers to paragraphs 123, 125 and 126.
18 Union of South Africa Official Reports and Papers, 1928, UG 35, Report of the Committee Appointed to the Inquiry into the Training of Natives in Medicine and Public Health (Loram), paras 63–72.
19 Rhodes University Cory Library Archives (henceforth: 'Rhodes, Cory'): MS 16, 575 Folder 1: SAIRR Conference on Medical Services for Non-Europeans and Training and Employment of Non-European and Rural Nurses held at Bloemfontein, 17 June 1932.
20 C. Rhodes, MS 16, 575 Folder 1: letter from Dr H. A. Moffat, Chair of committee to consider other forms of nurse training, sent to the Chairman of the Board, Johannesburg General Hospital, dated 6 September 1932.
21 NLS, D/86, Sulenkama correspondence.
22 M. Gelfand, *Christian Doctor and Nurse: The History of Medical Missions in South Africa From 1799–1976,* Sandton, RSA: Mariannhill Mission Press, 1984, pp. 174–7.
23 NLS, accession 7548, D/86, Sulenkama correspondence.
24 NLS, accession 7548, D/86, Sulenkama correspondence, letter from Marjorie Morrell, 30 September 1948.
25 NLS, accession 7548, D/86, Sulenkama correspondence.
26 S. Marks, ' "We were men nursing men" Male nursing on the mines in twentieth century South Africa', in W. Woodward, P. Hayes and G Minkley (eds), *Deep Histories. Gender and Colonialism in Southern Africa,* Amsterdam: Rodopi, 2002, pp. 177–205.

27   F. A. Swanson, '"Of unsound mind". A history of three Eastern Cape mental institutions, 1875–1910', unpublished MA thesis, University of Cape Town, c. 1977, pp. 147, 153.

28   S. Marks, *Not Either an Experimental Doll: the Separate Worlds of Three South African Women.* Pietermaritzburg: Killie Campbell Africana Library, University of Natal Press, 1987, p. 28.

29   J. Hyslop, 'Food, authority and politics: student riots in South African schools, 1945–1976' in S. Clingman (ed.), *Regions and Repertoires: Topics in South African Politics and Culture,* Johannesburg: 1991.

30   C. Rhodes, 1943–1970, Minutes of St Matthew's Mission College Council, April 1946–October 1960.

31   A. Mager, *Gender and the Making of a South African Bantustan. A Social History of the Transkei,* Oxford/Cape Town: 1999, pp. 197–205.

32   Marks, *Divided Sisterhood,* p. 107.

33   NLS, D/86, R. L. Paterson, The Nessie Knight Hospital, Sulenkama, 1949, Correspondence re. The threatened nurses' strike at Sulenkama, South Africa; R. L. Paterson, The Nessie Knight Hospital, Sulenkama, 1949, Report: Probationer nurses' threatened strike, 2–3 June 1949, South Africa; R. Paterson to Kerr, 20 June 1949.

34   NLS, D/86, R. Paterson to Kerr, 20 June 1949.

35   NLS, D/86, 'Particulars of the threatened strike, 2–3 June, 1949'.

36   A. D. Dodd, *Native Vocational Training,* Lovedale: 1938, p. 133.

37   NLS, D/86 'Particulars of the threatened strike, 2–3 June, 1949'.

38   Ibid.

39   Ibid.

40   NLS, D/86, Rough notes of an address to the nurses on 10 June 1949.

41   NLS, D/86, R. Paterson to Kerr, 20 June 1949.

42   Marks, *Divided Sisterhood,* p. 108.

43   Speech by Robert Sobukwe, quoted in Marks, *Divided Sisterhood,* p. 111.

44   Marks, *Divided Sisterhood,* pp. 109, 106–107, 157.

45   Mashaba, *Rising to the Challenge of Change,* p. 40.

46   Wellcome Archives SA/BMA/A.42: Letter from Leipoldt to Dr Cox, Secretary of the BMA, dated 1927.

47   B. Ka Mzolo, 'Nursing pioneers get recognition', *Natal Witness,* 2002 (19 April).

48   Marks, *Divided Sisterhood,* pp. 10, 196.

49   C. Hart, *Behind the Mask. Nurses, their Unions and Nursing Policy,* London: Bailliere Tindall, 1994, p. 1.

50   *Christian Express,* 1 February 1907, p. 30; Col. Sir E. N. Thornton, 'A medical and nursing service for natives in South Africa', *South African Medical Journal,* 1930, Vol. IV, (17), pp. 507–11.

51   Van Rensburg *et al. Health Care in South Africa,* p. 64.

52   Marks, *Divided Sisterhood,* pp. 115–33, 134.

53   L. M. Medlen, 'Ten nurse leaders and their contribution to the development of nursing in South Africa', unpublished M. Cur. Thesis, Department of Advanced Nursing Sciences, UNISA, Pretoria. 'Chapter 7, Alina W. Lekgetha', p. 113, refers to oral testimony of Mrs Lekgetha.

54   Ibid., p. 119. 'Baasskap' meaning domination, especially by whites, of other groups.

55   See also A. Digby and H. Sweet, 'Nurses as culture brokers in twentieth century South Africa', in W. Ernst (ed.), *Plural Medicine, Tradition and Modernity, 1800–2000,* London: Routledge.

56   H. W. Dyke, 'Training of African Nurses', *South African Medical Journal,* 1932, Vol. VI, pp. 546–9.

57   Quoted in Marks, *Divided Sisterhood,* p. 211. Mashaba, *Rising to the Challenge of Change,* p. 60, also refers to the 1960s and 1970s as a 'transitional stage of [cultural] development' for the Black nurse within her community, in which she had to exercise considerable diplomacy.

58   *Natal Witness,* 19 April 2002.

8　Health care and nursing coordination during the Nazi era in the region of Osnabrück

Mathilde Hackmann

Nursing in Nazi Germany has become a compelling topic in nursing history re-search since the 1980s. Alongside an increased interest in Nazi medicine among members of the medical profession, small groups of nurses have begun to in-vestigate the role of nursing during the Nazi era.[1] In particular, Hilde Steppe's thoughtful work on this topic has stimulated research in the field,[2] and today there is a growing body of literature. However, regional studies are rare, although such studies offer an opportunity to explore the detail of power relations that include nurses and nursing in the wider scheme of political and economic conditions within Nazi Germany. The value of regional investigations is well illustrated by Cornelia Rauh-Kühne;[3] her study of National Socialism in Catholic areas of Germany led her to conclude that the Nazis usually enjoyed less support from Catholic than from Protestant communities, but she also found strong regional differences. As nursing and nurse training was often closely associated with religious groups, it is very likely that these regional and religious differences will be reflected in nursing and health care. The main focus of this chapter is to determine the extent to which Nazi structures were integrated into health care and nursing within the region of Osnabrück (north-west Germany) and to assess the extent to which religious affiliation influenced these processes.

The state archives in Osnabrück were consulted to seek out sources for the study. The data that survive consist mainly of letters exchanged between the state and regional government with the local *Gesundheitsämter* (public health departments). A compendium of law relating to the health system was used to establish the legal context within which the letters were written. General statisti-cal information on the region of Osnabrück was also sought out. The findings were interpreted in the context of the published literature on nursing and welfare politics and the history of Osnabrück during the Nazi era.

Four case studies have been prepared to illustrate the impact of the *Gleichschaltung* (coordination) of services by the National Socialist (NS) gov-ernment on different aspects of health care and nursing. The chapter begins with a short account of the general situation in the region of Osnabrück, the local posi-tion in the administrative structure, and the broad position of nursing and health care during the Nazi era.

THE REGION OF OSNABRÜCK

The region of Osnabrück (*Regierungsbezirk*) covered the north-west part of Germany next to the Dutch border. The region supported 516,447 inhabitants in 1939,[4] 100,000 of these citizens living in the largest city of Osnabrück. The region was principally agricultural but there were some industrial centres. Fifty-five per cent of the inhabitants were Catholic; most of the remainder of the population was Protestant. In general terms, regional differences in religion have been noted to have a considerable impact on political parties, and in the Catholic areas of Osnabrück the NSDAP (Nazi Party) did not win elections before 1933. However, when the Nazis came to power nationally in 1933 their influence began to extend even to Catholic regions. The increasing influence of NS ideology on local society in Osnabrück can be illustrated by the successful development of concentration camps in the western part of the region. These camps were a new departure, first introduced by the Nazi government to house political prisoners from the German population; later, foreign slave labourers were forced to work in German industries.[5] Here in *Emsland*, where there was a predominantly Catholic population, Elke Suhr argues that promises of work, economic prosperity and a rise in national status for the whole region influenced the views of individuals, the wider community, regional organizations, the press and even the church, and persuaded them to come to terms with this feature of fascism.[6]

STRUCTURE OF GOVERNMENT DURING THE NAZI ERA

Although it is often assumed that the Nazi Party exercised governmental control as soon as it gained power, in reality the process was far more complex. Throughout the Nazi era, there was always a dual structure of power. On the one hand, there was a formal bureaucratic structure designed to manage and administer the state, while on the other hand was the party structure. When the Nazis came to power in 1933, they set out to destroy democratic structures in a number of ways. Party members were put in control of key organizations such as the police; the *Länder* parliaments were abolished; and *Gleichschaltung* (coordination) was introduced to all organizations. This meant that many organizations were restructured or even disbanded. The policy was particularly directed at political parties and trade unions. Another strategy employed by the Nazis was to place active party members in administrative positions; in effect, such a strategy might result in individuals assuming a dual administrative and political role. However, this strategy was not always successful and hierarchies were often unclear. Jane Caplan describes this situation as follows:

> Rival hierarchies, competing agencies, uncertain chains of command, duplication of responsibilities, reluctant pooling of information, inadequate machinery for coordination – these are typical symptoms of the administrative incoherence which now constitutes the most familiar picture of government in the Third Reich.[7]

Eckhard Hansen,[8] studying the welfare politics of the NS state, views this administrative incoherence as putting the NS idea of the 'survival of the fittest' into its own governmental structure. Although this might be too generalized a view, it is evident that such a dual structure had potential consequences for the organization of health care and nursing.

The region of Osnabrück was a part of the administrative province of Hanover, one of the eleven provinces of the former *Land* of Prussia. Because the Nazis abolished the *Länder* parliaments, the region of Osnabrück was directly responsible to and under the control of the Home Office in Berlin. The organization of the NSDAP (Nazi party) consisted of sections or *Gaue*. These *Gaue* did not necessarily cover the same geographical areas as the governmental units. For example, the *Gau Weser-Ems* included the region of Osnabrück, the *Land* Oldenburg and the city of Bremen (Figure 8.1).

The power of the NSDAP and its influence on local government was dependent on the so-called *Gauleiter* (party district leader). The *Gauleiter* of the *Gau Weser-*

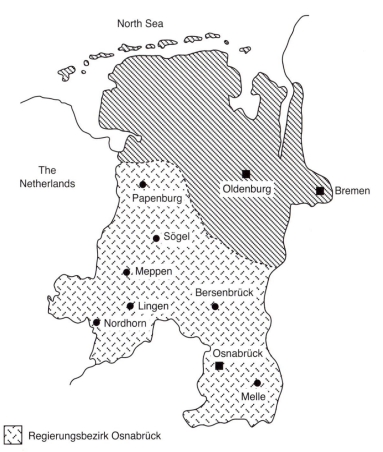

Figure 8.1   Map of the region of Osnabrück.

Ems region, Karl Röver, had been a party member since 1925 and is described as one with a ' . . . certain critical distance from many of the unpleasant phenomena of German home politics in the NS system'.[9] So it might be expected that the power of the party in the region of Osnabrück was not as strong as in other areas.

HEALTH CARE AND NURSING

The German welfare system that had expanded during the Weimar Republic and the world economic crisis did not fit with the NS ideology. The Weimar system had sought to increase services for the whole population, for example by introducing unemployment benefits and reforms for workers and pensioners.[10] By contrast, the underlying idea of NS welfare as described by Thomas E. J. de Witt was that:

> Ultimately welfare would become obsolete, since the Nazis interpreted poverty as primarily a racial problem which could be solved through preventive health care and economic assistance for the racially valuable – and politically reliable – citizen therefore precluding welfare dependency.[11]

As a result, new laws were introduced and responsibility for welfare was transferred to the individual. The existing system of health care, a system that included compulsory healthcare insurance, did not change but the self-government of the healthcare insurance companies was eliminated.[12]

In 1934, under the NS government, so-called *Gesundheitsämter* (public health departments) were established to introduce and supervise health promotion, and by 1938 there were 744 *Gesundheitsämter* in Germany.[13] Their principal focus was to standardize and regulate nationwide state implementation of NS eugenics. In practice, various new laws supported this policy and gave the physicians of the *Gesundheitsämter* the power to control matters of public health; for example, these physicians issued the eugenic certificate that was required before marriage.

Another method used to introduce the Nazi ideology into the practice of health and social care was the establishment of the NSV (*Nationalsozialistische Volkswohlfahrt* or NS People's Welfare Organization). This new organization was developed as an addition to existing welfare agencies run by the Catholic or Protestant church and some other public and private organizations. The new organization employed its own nurses and rapidly assumed greater importance than the older agencies because state money was granted more generously to the NSV. The result of these moves was that, although the NSV managed to take over increased responsibilities in health and social care, there were always problems in achieving cooperation with other institutions.[14] Asmus Nitschke, who studied public health in Bremen during the Nazi era, concluded that 'the much vaunted "thriving cooperation" between all NSV organizations and the public health departments was obviously only a pipe-dream'.[15] The main focus of the NSV became the care of small children; consequently, the role of district or community nurses now assumed new significance as they were expected to have the greatest opportunity to influence the population.[16] However, as with other governmental reforms, there were regional differences in the implementation of this policy and the chronic shortage of qualified nurses ensured that the NSV never succeeded in taking over all the district nursing services run by the churches.[17,18]

When the Nazis came to power, German nurses were not well organized. In 1928 about 50 per cent of all nurses were organized in Catholic and Protestant nursing associations. These associations included not only nuns and deaconesses living under strict regulations but also secular nurses. Nursing associations, which were sometimes called sisterhoods, organized continuing professional education and offered jobs to nurses. Sometimes a nursing association was responsible for organizing the nursing service in hospitals. Beside religious-oriented nursing associations, a number of secular nursing associations attracted nurses, the Red Cross Nursing Association being one of the most popular. Significantly, there was no national association dedicated to supporting the interests of all nurses. The lack of a unifying national system weakened the position of nurses. In addition to lacking a national voice, the position of nurses was further undermined by the fact that most of them were female and, in a gendered world, had a relatively low status. Professional skills were often confused with personal characteristics. Steppe concludes that these were the 'classical problems of nursing'.[19]

The NSV also established a Nazi nursing sisterhood and was given control over all nursing associations by the government. This move was particularly important as the nursing associations, secular and religious, made a substantial contribution to the number of students who completed their training each year and became trained nurses. Perhaps most significant of all, the government established new rules for nurse training in the Nursing Act of 1938. These new rules included a requirement that nurses be instructed in eugenic principles. An unexpected consequence of all this official interest in nursing was to raise the status of nursing in the eyes of the general population. This change was welcomed by many nurses, and might have influenced their views of the NS state.[20]

Four case studies that centre on nursing issues within the region of Osnabrück follow. These explore the extent that NS influence impacted on the health care of the region and illustrate some of the tensions that were created.

NATIONAL SOCIALIST COORDINATION IN THE REGION OF OSNABRÜCK

Introduction of *Gesundheitsämter* (public health departments)

Before the law of 1934, a network of formalized public health provision had existed in Germany with various regional differences. The new law was intended to secure the coordination of all health services and demanded the universal introduction of public health departments. In some regions – for example, Prussia, of which Osnabrück had formed a part – public health departments had been in place in the cities from the nineteenth century. That established system had also included the appointment of *Kreisärzte* (physicians with public health duties) in rural areas. In the city of Osnabrück, 1934 saw the existing public health department integrated into the new structure. The various *Kreisärzte* in the region were also absorbed and public health departments were established in each of the nine *Kreis* or local administrative units.[21]

The surviving records of the public health departments in the region of Osnabrück suggest that integration of the departments was accomplished in 1938; there is certainly evidence that the former public health department of the city of Osnabrück was restructured between 1936 and 1938.[22] The premises of the public health department changed and staff formerly employed by the city now worked in the new institution, which served a wider area. The new public health departments continued the traditional tasks of preventative health care such as tuberculosis welfare, family welfare and school health, but they also had an important new role of social control. Their new primary objective was to implement NS eugenic policies; that is to build up genetic files on all people and seek to control their reproduction. No evidence has been traced to indicate whether this policy objective was successfully achieved in Osnabrück.

Community or district nurses might be expected to assume a significant role in the implementation of this eugenic policy by the public health department. The patchy nature of the surviving sources makes it difficult to trace the extent of the influence of the nurses, to determine their commitment to this eugenic objective or to reconstruct their activities. The names of fourteen 'public health' nurses survive in a list prepared in Osnabrück in 1938. 'Public health' nurses had received training in social work in addition to their nursing training. These nurses worked in the city, had direct access to families and were well placed to collect information. Of the fourteen nurses listed, ten worked as family social workers, one of whom specialized in infant care, two worked as tuberculosis nurses, one worked with adolescents and one with people suffering from venereal diseases.

Although there is little evidence to illustrate the daily work of the nurses, two travel diaries written by public health nurses from the *Kreis* Lingen provide some data. An extract from the travel diary of one of these public health nurses (Table 8.1) demonstrates the time she spent on home visits,[23] an activity that might offer an opportunity to control or influence her client group. She was certainly conscientious and committed to her duties. Even in the cold month of November, she visited people at home by bicycle on ten days. It is very likely that the nurse took notes following her visits, but it is unclear how much of this information was added to the genetic files of her clients that were created by the department. However, we do know that an effort was made to train public health nurses in eugenics. The diary of another nurse records her attendance at an eight-day course on racial politics in Cologne in July 1936.[24] This seems to be part of an organized endeavour to train nurses in eugenics and gain their support for the Nazi ideology.

Although the surviving sources from Osnabrück and *Kreis* Lingen provide only a patchy account of the role of public health nurses in the region, they do demonstrate that the public health department made positive efforts to educate

Table 8.1 Travel diary of the public health nurse Schweigmann for the month of November 1937

Date	Time	Route	Daily allowance/travelling expenses	Kilometres
2.11.1937	08:00–13:00	Biene, home visits		14
4.11.1937	08:00–13:00	Bicycle Wachendorf, home visit		14
5.11.1937	07:14–18:00	Train to Salzbergen, travel home by bicycle	0.5 RM, expenses 1.30 RM	26
9.11.1937	08:00–13:00	Bicycle Laxten, home visits		5
12.11.1937	08:00–13:00	Bicycle Bawinkel, home visits	0.5 RM	20
13.11.1937	08:00–12:00	Bicycle Biene, home visits		14
15.11.1937	07:14–12:45	By train to Salzbergen, home visits	Expenses 2.00 RM	
23.11.1937	08:00–13:00	Bicycle Schepsdorf, home visits		4
24.11.1937	08:00–13:00	Bicycle Darme, home visits		4
26.11.1937	07:14–17:20	By train to Salzbergen, home visits	0.5 RM, expenses 2.00 RM	
30.11.1937	08:00–13:00	Bicycle Bienerfeld, home visits		18

Source: Staatsarchiv Osnabrück REP 630 Lin Nr. 39 Reisetagebuch der Gesundheitspflegerin Schweigmann 1935–38.
Note: RM = Reichsmark.

nurses and strengthen their commitment to the approved ideologies. It is not possible to conclude with certainty that nurses became active and willing instruments of the Nazi health philosophy; it is equally impossible to reject this possibility. This is particularly so in a region that was able to tolerate the setting up of concentration camps despite the presence of a large Catholic population. Similarly, willing complicity with official directives is a real possibility among the members of a traditionally low-status profession that was enjoying flattering attention from those who held power.

The influence of the Nazi laws on nurse education

It has been suggested that the status and educational position of nurses might have impacted on their response and contribution to NS public health. A second important issue will now be explored, which might contribute to an understanding of the position of nurses in the region of Osnabrück – their education. Nurse education was not high on the agenda when the Nazis came to power. According to the compendium of law, a number of new laws concerning public health were passed between 1934 and 1937. However, no new laws affecting nurse education were passed in this period.[25] Nurse education did not attract significant attention until 1938. The changes that were then introduced can be attributed to a concern about the shortage of nurses. This was first officially expressed in 1937 as an issue to be addressed. It became particularly urgent as a part of the preparations for war.[26]

The position of nurses and nursing was particularly vulnerable in the context of NS philosophy. This followed from the Nazi concern to encourage and nurture an expanding and healthy population. To support this policy, women were encouraged to marry early and, on marriage, were awarded a state grant to help establish a household. As the majority of nurses were women, this policy encouraged short working careers for nurses and contributed to the national shortage. In response to this situation, campaigns to recruit more nurses were initiated in 1937.[27]

One of the efforts to meet the shortage of nurses was the establishment of new nursing schools. The government in Berlin wanted to establish nursing schools in all public hospitals with at least 100 beds where there were enough 'competent teaching doctors'.[28] It was calculated that one student nurse could be trained for every ten hospital beds; thus if a hospital had 150 beds the school could accept fifteen student nurses. The proposed formula also stated that one-fifth of all trained nurses could be replaced by student nurses, and two student nurses could replace one trained nurse.

In June 1937 only two schools of nursing, both situated in the city of Osnabrück, existed in the whole region. That month all hospitals in the region of Osnabrück were assessed for their suitability as locations for new schools of nursing.[29] The survey of hospitals, beds and nurses revealed a complicated situation.

There were six hospitals of 100 beds or more. Of the six only three were state run; churches or private institutions ran the remainder. One of the state-run hospitals (Landes-Heil and Pflegeanstalt Osnabrück) was a psychiatric hospital, which claimed that no trained nurses were employed. There was indeed no recognized formal training programme for the preparation of psychiatric nurses in Germany. However, an apprenticeship model was widely applied that was designed to introduce recruits to patient care. It seems very likely that at least some of the 129 'other personnel' mentioned in the report would have been these informally educated 'nurses'. A second state-run hospital (*Städtische Krankenanstalten* with 575 beds) already had a nursing school with forty-one student nurses. It was proposed that a new nursing school be set up in the third state hospital and the fate of this school will form the third case study in this chapter. The remaining forty-nine hospitals, which housed a total of approximately 3,700 beds, were too small to accommodate a school and often did not have a doctor on the permanent staff.

In addition to seeking an increase in the numbers of nurses in training, the NS government was concerned to introduce Nazi ideology and eugenics to nurse education. Before the surge of interest in nurse training managed by the NS government, few nursing texts had been available and it was common for student nurses to study without the use of textbooks. An official book for nurse education had been available for some time but, after the tenth edition was published in 1928, almost a decade lapsed before a new edition appeared under the NS government. The eleventh edition of this official textbook was published in 1937; in this edition, sections on Nazi ideology and eugenics were introduced. These sections were extended in the twelfth edition of 1938, at the same time as use of the book was made compulsory in all training establishments.[30] It can be confirmed that within the region of Osnabrück, books for the schools of nursing were purchased through the government and the nurses' examinations tested knowledge of the contents of this text including the eugenics sections.[31]

The Nursing Act of 1938 included other significant requirements. The length of training was specified and, very significantly, the personal characteristics of students and members of the examination boards were spelled out. Students and examiners must be Aryan. It was possible to establish special nursing schools for Jews but this did not occur in the region of Osnabrück as there was only a very small Jewish community and no Jewish hospital.

These strategies made little immediate impression on the problem of recruiting nurses, and one year after the new Nurses Act, the government was sufficiently exercised by the problem of nurse recruitment and nurse education to undertake the second national survey of schools of nursing in two years. In addition to gathering information, this exercise sought to supervise and encourage the reforms. Schools were asked questions that confirmed the administration's priorities for nurses and nurse training:[32]

1 Is suitable accommodation available for student nurses?
2 Who will give the lectures on the 'world view'?[33] Has this teacher been appointed in agreement with the party member responsible for training?
3 Who is responsible for regular physical training?

It appears that in at least some settings the monitoring of nurse education was taken seriously and was carried out with care. A book published to commemorate the seventh-fifth anniversary of the nursing school at the Marienhospital Osnabrück mentions that approval of the school as a training institution in 1939 was only renewed when all three questions were answered to the government's satisfaction.[34] In this Catholic hospital, it was well recognized that the school had to meet the special requirements for its existence to continue.

The importance of the nurse as an 'official' representative with legitimate access to private homes made her an obvious object of interest to a state that was concerned with eugenic regulation of the population. Although nursing was virtually ignored in the early years of NS rule, by 1937 the vigorous efforts made by the administration were designed to pull the divided occupation of nursing into the NS sphere of influence. In the region of Osnabrück, at least some of these efforts appear to have been regarded as successful by at least some observers, those who recorded data relating to the Marienhospital for example. However, the continued existence of many smaller hospitals and the complexities of care provision suggest that many areas of nursing and health care were not easily accessible to these direct government interventions.

The establishment of a school of nursing at the *Kreiskrankenhaus* (district hospital) in Nordhorn

The thrust to increase the numbers of trained nurses was taken very seriously in some locations and in 1938 the *Landrat* (executive of the local government) of the *Kreis* Grafschaft Bentheim asked the regional government in Osnabrück to establish a school of nursing at the district hospital in Nordhorn.[35] The first approach with this request was rejected because the regional government did not consider the existing buildings suitable. They specified that the operating theatre be rebuilt and that the hospital should provide evidence of proper staff accommodation. After the modifications had been made, the application was submitted to the Home Office in Berlin and the school was officially approved in August 1938. Local records suggest that twelve student nurses belonging to the Nazi sisterhood of the NSV Oldenburg had already been recruited and had begun their training in spring 1938. These students completed their eighteen-month training in the autumn of 1939. The project to establish this school encountered repeated problems, one of which was the lack of sufficient trained nurses to supervise students on the wards. This clinical and professional concern was set aside, perhaps under pressure to ensure the survival and success of the school. Another problem was regarded more seriously and delayed the approval of the school examination board until February 1939. This was the difficulty experienced in confirming the Aryan ancestry of the medical director's wife. The inadequate numbers of qualified nurses might be ignored but there was no question regarding the racial requirements of the NS regulations. It was essential that they were respected and complied with.

In spring 1939, the local government applied for additional central funding because the school was experiencing financial problems. This became the subject of a number of letters between the *Landrat* (regional government) and the Home

Office in Berlin. This correspondence continued until April 1941. The *Kreis* wanted to close the school because it was so short of funds. This option was rejected under the strict laws of the Nazi regime. One practical problem was that the *Kreis* had engaged additional personnel to assist with the training of student nurses without the agreement of the regional government in Osnabrück. The Home Office in Berlin argued that these costs were unnecessary. In the end, a compromise was agreed; nurse education was to be discontinued during the war years. It seems that the Home Office permitted this only because the NSV Oldenburg was not prepared to send new student nurses to the school in 1941.

This situation is open to several interpretations. The local hospital administration might have come to lack commitment to the project for many reasons. The picture painted so far of the nursing school in Nordhorn has been constructed principally from surviving regional archival sources. A slightly different picture of the school emerges when the official statistical list of nursing schools in Germany, published centrally in 1941 by the Home Office in Berlin, is examined.[36] This confirmed the number of student nurses as twelve. However, the students recorded in the local sources as members of the Nazi sisterhood were described in the report from Berlin as members of the Protestant Association of Nurses. This statement, made by those who were viewing the situation from afar, is possibly not surprising because the qualified nurses in the Nordhorn hospital were Protestant deaconesses. This feature of the records might mask a very complicated situation where tensions were heightened in a public hospital, staffed by deaconesses, when these women were required to use the official nursing textbook and cooperate in the education of student nurses who were members of the Nazi sisterhood. If the deaconess nurses were unwilling to engage wholeheartedly with this project, the hospital managers might have been pressured into incurring additional expenses to support the programme. Whatever the reasons behind the lack of success of the Nordhorn project, the existence within the scheme of different and potentially opposed ideologies was very likely to undermine such a project.

This case study, of the school of nursing in Nordhorn, is an example of the failure of NS coordination. Although the system managed to control the exam board members, it failed to establish the new school. However, the final compromise that stopped nurse education during the war years meant that none of the parties involved lost face.

Coordination of the care of pregnant women, infants and small children

The NS preoccupation with the creation of a large, healthy, Aryan population meant that much of their interest was focused on the care of pregnant women, infants and small children. In an effort to reduce infant mortality, midwives were required to make quarterly visits to infants during the first year of their lives. Extra funding was made available to support this policy, a commitment that confirmed the priorities of the state. Midwives were paid five Reichsmark for each infant they supervised and monitored during the first life year.[37]

The NSV, or party welfare organization, was particularly interested in the welfare of the healthy part of the population and in the promotion of health rather than in the care of the sick and disabled. As a result, attention was increasingly directed to child welfare clinics. Initially, public health departments controlled all child care. However, this proved to be problematic in practice and in 1941 all child welfare clinics in Germany were officially transferred to the NSV.[38] In the region of Osnabrück, all public health departments were required to deliver lists to the regional government of the number of clinics in the region. They were also required to state to what degree NSV nurses, NSV infant nurses and NSV social workers were involved in the work of clinics. The lists clearly show regional differences. On the whole, NSV staff were scarcely involved in the region of Osnabrück.[39] It seems that, before this survey, child welfare clinics in Osnabrück were managed with little direct interference by the NSV. This might indicate that NS ideas were not influential locally. However, it is possible to argue a different case. Surviving records cannot indicate how far NS ideology penetrated into the workings of the clinics under the influence of the midwives and other personnel employed in them. It could be that the position in Osnabrück, without direct NSV intervention, was sympathetic to NS ideology and that the professionals engaged in the clinics supported this position. If this were the case, central and local NS supporters might be content to tolerate a position that did not permit direct intervention. The scanty nature of the surviving records makes a more accurate interpretation of this situation extremely difficult.

The region of *Kreis* Aschendorf in the northern part of Osnabrück appears to have been something of a special case. Infant mortality during the first year of life, recorded as 10.6 per cent in 1942, was the second highest figure in the region. This problem persisted even though child welfare clinics had been expanded since the late 1930s.[40] Further efforts were made in 1940 to expand the number of child welfare clinics in this *Kreis* – from thirty to fifty – by appointing eleven new nurses. These new nurses included three public health nurses from the public health department in Aschendorf and the introduction of six district nurses. Sixteen midwives in the area were also involved and were awarded extra funding.[41] These changes occurred in spite of what Hansen describes as the lack of trained staff, which was the most serious problem preventing the expansion of NSV activities in nursing and health.[42] This willingness to commit funds at a financially difficult time suggests that there was some commitment to the NS wish to support infant welfare even when clinics were not directly under the control of the NSV. Three years later, in 1943, the sixteen midwives in the *Kreis* Aschendorf with a special contract for running child welfare clinics were reduced to eight.[43] At this later date, it was argued that the NSV would run all child welfare clinics with their own personnel.

The literature suggests that the involvement of different services in the welfare clinics caused confusion and might result in double visits and other wasteful duplication of effort.[44] This problem is not immediately visible in the records for the region of Osnabrück. Detailed regulations were created to manage cooperation between the NSV and the public health departments in the field of child health

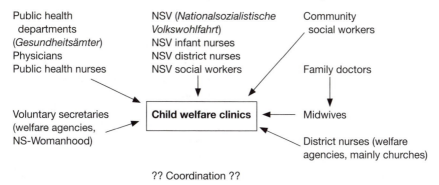

Figure 8.2 Parties involved in the care of pregnant women, infants and small children.

care. A local decree published in 1941 advised nurses and social workers responsible for child welfare on how to cooperate with the doctors and other personnel in the public health departments.[45] The number of individuals involved illustrates something of the complexity of the situation in child welfare clinics. Figure 8.2 suggests that many complex additional problems might be experienced when attempting to coordinate the various groups. Although the NSV was expected to run all child welfare clinics from 1943, it did not have the personnel or the funding to achieve this task without the cooperation of other organizations. The desired unified and united child welfare service was not something that could be readily achieved and the familiar problems of duplication of efforts and activities continued.

CONCLUSION

This study has been limited by the uneven nature of the surviving records. Many records were destroyed during the Second World War. Perhaps the most abiding conclusion is of the number and complexity of the influences that affected health care. Apparently coherent central policies and directives became ever more complex as attempts were made to implement them among a population whose response was affected by personal differences of belief and ideology. The much-vaunted strategy of NS *Gleichschaltung* (coordination) worked in some parts of the healthcare system but failed in others, and it is not always possible to be sure why this occurred. The introduction of *Gesundheitsämter* appears to have been achieved very quickly, in part because the existing public health system could readily be assimilated. The question of how far the system achieved its goal of controlling people is more difficult to answer. It has been possible to cite one instance in Nordhorn where the process of founding a new school of nursing was held up until the Aryan antecedents of a key person were confirmed. However, when the school in question ultimately foundered, the scraps of evidence that survive suggest that divisions and differences of belief confounded the process of educating Nazi nurses in this public hospital staffed by Protestant nurses.

The reforms in nurse education were implemented in the region. But this did not prove to be a simple process that produced large numbers of suitably trained nurses. The experiences of those attempting to found the new school of nursing in Nordhorn seem to be particularly instructive. Considerable effort was invested to found the school. It appears that a conscious attempt was made to graft a school in the new traditions of the Nazi sisterhood onto an institution that was grounded in the Protestant deaconess tradition. This failed and it might be that the disparate nature of German nursing, with no experience of a national system of organization in the period before 1933, condemned the imposition of a more centralized system to failure. In the provincial hospitals, deaconess orders and sisterhoods were accustomed to managing their own affairs and were well acquainted with ways of continuing their independence.

The problems in the cooperation among the various parties involved in the care of pregnant women, infants and small children have proved to be immensely complex. In the Osnabrück region, the NSV appeared to concentrate its attention in *Kreis* Aschendorf where the problems appeared greatest; other parts of the region received less attention. Even this selective approach, however, was not a reflection of a planned and economic division of activities as duplication of effort was still likely to occur.

The overwhelming impression of health care in the region is of considerable potential for confusion as an attempt was made to impose an approved set of NS values and priorities upon the health care system in a complex region where a range of values and beliefs was deeply embedded in existing structures and practitioners.

NOTES

1   H. Steppe, F. Koch, H. Weisbrod-Frey, *Krankenpflege im Nationalsozialismus*, Frankfurt: Mabuse-Verlag, 1986.
2   J. Dornheim, U. Greb, 'Theoretische Ansätze zur Diskussion über die Beteiligung von Krankenpflegepersonal an den Patientenmorden im Nationalsozialismus', in O. Niethammer (ed.), *Frauen und Nationalsozialismus – Historische und kulturgeschichtliche Positionen*, Osnabrück: Unversitätsverlag Rasch, 1996, pp. 10–23.
3   C. Rauh-Kühne, 'Katholisches Sozialmilieu, Region und Nationalsozialismus', in H. Möller, A. Wirsching and W. Ziegler (eds), *Nationalsozialismus in der Region, Sondernummer Schriftenreihe der Vierteljahreshefte für Zeitgeschichte*, München: Oldenbourg, 1996, pp. 213–35.
4   G. Steinwascher, *Gestapo Osnabrück meldet . . . Polizei- und Regierungsberichte aus dem Regierungsbezirk Osnabrück aus den Jahren 1933 bis 1936*, Osnabrück: Selbstverlag des Vereins für Geschichte und Landeskunde von Osnabrück, 1995.
5   B. J. Wendt, *Das nationalsozialistische Deutschland, Beiträge zur Politik und Zeitgeschichte*, Opladen: Leske & Budrich, 2000.
6   E. Suhr, *Die Emslandlager: Die politische und wirtschaftliche Bedeutung der emsländischen Konzentrations- und Strafgefangenenlager 1933–1945*, Bremen: Donat und Temmen, 1985.
7   J. Caplan, 'Bureaucracy, politics and the national socialist state', in P. D. Stachura (ed.), *The Shaping of the Nazi State*, London: Croom Helm, 1978, pp. 234–56, quotation p. 234.

8   E. Hansen, *Wohlfahrtspolitik im NS-Staat – Motivationen, Konflikte und Machtstrukturen im, Sozialismus der Tat' des Dritten Reiches*, Augsburg: Maro Verlag, 1991.

9   P. Hüttenberger, *Die Gauleiter – Studie zum Wandel des Machgefüges in der NSDAP, Schriftenreihe der Vierteljahreshefte für Zeitgeschichte*, Stuttgart: Deutsche Verlags-Anstalt, 1969, p. 197.

10 M. G. Schmidt, *Sozialpolitik in Deutschland. Historische Entwicklung und internationaler Vergleich*, 2nd edn, Opladen: Leske & Budrich, 1998.

11 T. E. J. de Witt, 'The economics and politics of welfare in the Third Reich', *Central European History*, 1978, Vol. 11, p. 260.

12 S. Leibfried und F. Tennstedt, *Berufsverbote und Sozialpolitik 1933 – die Auswirkungen der nationalsozialistischen Machtergreifung auf die Krankenkassenverwaltung und die Kassenärzte*, 3rd edn, Bremen: Universität Bremen, Presse- und Informationsdienst, 1981.

13 A. Labisch und F. Tennstedt, 'Gesundheitsamt oder Amt für Volksgesundheit? Zur Entwicklung des öffentlichen Gesundheitswesens seit 1933', in N. Frei (ed.), *Medizin und Gesundheitspolitik in der NS-Zeit*, München: Oldenbourg Verlag, 1991, pp. 35–66.

14 Hansen, *Wohlfahrtspolitik*.

15 A. Nitschke, *Die ,Erbpolizei' im Nationalsozialismus – Zur Alltagsgeschichte der Gesundheitsämter im Dritten Reich*, Opladen/Wiesbaden: Westdeutscher Verlag, 1999, p. 48.

16 H. Steppe, 'Nursing in Nazi Germany', *Western Journal of Nursing Research*, 1992, Vol. 14, pp. 744–53.

17 Hansen, *Wohlfahrtspolitik*.

18 C. Sachße und F. Tennstedt, *Der Wohlfahrtsstaat im Nationalsozialismus – Geschichte der Armenfürsorge in Deutschland Band 3*, Stuttgart: Kohlhammer, 1992.

19 H. Steppe, 'Krankenpflege bis 1933', in Steppe (ed.), *Krankenpflege im Nationalsozialismus*, Frankfurt a. Main: Mabuse-Verlag, 1996, pp. 33–59, quotation p. 54.

20 Steppe, *Krankenpflege im Nationalsozialismus*.

21 StAOS REP 430 Dez 3003 Akz. 19/56 Nr. 222 Betreuung für Säuglinge und Kleinkinder 1928–1945.

22 StAOS REP 430 Dez 303 acc 15/65 Nr. 9 Geschäftsräume des Gesundheitsamtes Kreis Osnabrück-Stadt.

23 StAOS REP 630 Lin Nr. 39 Reisetagebuch der Gesundheitspflegerin Schweigmann 1935–1938.

24 StAOS REP 630 Lin Nr. 40 Tagebuch Waldschmidt.

25 Reichsgesetzblatt, Ministerialblatt für die Preußische innere Verwaltung 1933–1935, Ministerial-Blatt des Reichs- und Preußischen Ministerium des Innern 1936–1943, Berlin.

26 D. Duesterberg, 'Pflege im Zweiten Weltkrieg', in H. Steppe (ed.), *Krankenpflege im Nationalsozialismus*, Frankfurt a. Main: Mabuse-Verlag, 1996, pp. 119–34.

27 Ibid.

28 StAOS REP 430–303–38/76 Nr. 3 Ausbildung von Krankenpflegepersonal 1933–57.

29 StAOS Ausbildung von Krankenpflegepersonal 1933–1957.

30 K. Döhne, R. Bauernfeind, 'Krankenpflegelehrbücher im Nationalsozialismus', unpublished typescript, Frankfurt am Main: Berufsfortbildungswerk des DGB, 1984.

31 StAOS REP 430 Dez 303 Akz. 19/56 Nr. 5 Einrichtung und Personalausstattung von Krankenpflegeschulen 1937–1948.

32 StAOS Einrichtung und Personalausstattung von Krankenpflegeschulen 1937–1948.

33 'World view' was a concept created by Adolf Hitler, the leader of the Nazi party. It was not well defined but can be seen as a consistent construct of ideas of the NS

ideology. B. J. Wendt, *Deutschland 1933–1945, Das "Dritte Reich" Handbuch zur Geschichte*, Hannover: Fackelträger-Verlag, 1995.

34   Marienhospital Osnabrück, *75 Jahre Krankenpflegeschule am Marienhospital Osnabrück 1920–1995*, Osnabrück: Druck- und Verlagshaus Fromm, 1995.

35   StAOS Einrichtung und Personalausstattung von Krankenpflegeschulen 1937–1948

36   Ministerialblatt des Reichs- und Preußischen Ministeriums des Innern, 1941, Nr. 27, 1192i–1192pp.

37   StAOS Betreuung für Säuglinge und Kleinkinder 1928–1945.

38   Hansen, *Wohlfahrtspolitik*.

39   StAOS Betreuung für Säuglinge und Kleinkinder 1928–1945.

40   Ibid.

41   Ibid.

42   Hansen, *Wohlfahrtspolitik*.

43   StAOS REP 630 Asch NR. 308 Einschaltung der Hebammen in die Schwangeren-, Säuglings- und Kleinkinderfürsorge.

44   Hansen, *Wohlfahrtspolitik*.

45   StAOS Betreuung für Säuglinge und Kleinkinder 1928–1945.

9 'In England we did nursing'

Caribbean and British nurses in Great Britain and Canada, 1950–70

Margaret Shkimba and Karen Flynn

In the aftermath of the Second World War, the supply of trained nurses available for work fell far short of the demand for their services. This shortage can be attributed to various influences; however, an increased demand in industrializing countries for institutional nurses, high occupational attrition and competition for women labourers from other, more attractive, occupations were prominent causal factors. Owing to the nursing shortage, efforts to induce young women into the profession were pursued through many channels and in many countries. This proved beneficial for thousands of young women by offering to them the opportunity to enter into a career that provided them with a skilled education, certain employment and the chance to travel to countries around the world. Both Canada and the UK experienced chronic shortages in their nursing workforce and for both countries part of the solution appeared in the form of immigrant nursing labour; nurses went in sizeable numbers from the Caribbean to the UK, and from the Caribbean and the UK to Canada.

This chapter seeks to chart the migration experiences of young black Caribbean and white British women who trained in the UK and who subsequently emigrated as nurses to Canada. Through our separate research, we sought answers to similar questions. Why choose nursing as an occupation? What was the impetus behind migration? And for Caribbean nurses, why Britain and then Canada? We were especially interested in the immigrant nurses' perceptions of the professional transition, and in what strategies these nurses used to cope with their new country and working environment.

This study is based on oral interviews with nurses who emigrated to Canada from the Caribbean and the UK after the Second World War, between 1950 and 1970. Many of the nurses interviewed lived in southern Ontario, an area that hosts the largest urban population in Canada. For this study, the interviews of ten black Caribbean-born and twelve white British-born nurses are used.[1] The interviews were conducted between 1995 and 2002, at which time the subjects had an age range of between sixty and eighty-five. This research provides insight into the migration process as experienced by black and white, professional, young women. What is seen are the nuances of both inter- and intra-race relations, particularly as applicable to gender (young women) and occupation (nurses). The following major topics for analysis emerged from this research: how is it that despite living in a racist society, and against the backdrop of racialized public discourses surrounding immigration restrictions, the experiences of the Caribbean nurses, both in their British and Canadian migrations, are not remembered as particularly racist? Second, why is it that white British nurses, despite official status in Canada as a most favoured immigrant group enjoying close cultural and ethnic similarities, felt alienated and isolated within the predominantly white Canadian workplace? Indeed, these sentiments are similar to the words of Caribbean nurses; each group faced the experienced of being 'othered', albeit in different ways. We argue that it was their common identity as nurses, particularly as nurses who trained in the UK, which served to mediate their experiences of racial and cultural disunity, in Britain for the Caribbean nurses, and in Canada for both the Caribbean and British nurses.

This common identity experienced by the two sets of nurses was acquired during training and, therefore, under vulnerable circumstances; that is, during a particular age (young adulthood), in an environment away from home, living in shared accommodation, biding by the same rules, learning the same skills and situated firmly within an established hierarchy. For very many of the women, it was their first time away from home, and not all who entered training stayed to finish. One British nurse spent her first year in Preliminary Training at a converted country mansion in Dewsbury. She recalled: '[an] Irish girl was terribly, terribly homesick . . . she cried and cried. She cried buckets full. In the end she just went back home again, she just couldn't stand being away from home.'[2] Wastage rates were high throughout this period.[3]

Accounts of British women's immigration to Canada in the post-war period have emphasized the experiences of war brides, which situated female migration within the family context.[4] Studies that explore the migration of Caribbean peoples tend to focus on migrant farm and domestic workers, with an emphasis on race and racism.[5] Migrant nurses were a large and significant element within post-war professional migration. In 1962, nurses made up 20 per cent of immigrants with an occupation classified as 'professional'.[6] In raising this topic, for two select groups of nurses, we hope to encourage the study of the phenomenon. We also hope to contribute to the understanding of nursing in both Canada and Britain as told through the voices of those previously silent in nursing scholarship.

TRAINING, EDUCATION AND IDENTITY FORMATION

Although their occupational choices were shaped by gender expectations, which, in turn, had already limited educational pursuits, for most women in the post-war era there was an expectation to work, at least for the period between school leaving and marriage. For black women in the Caribbean, there were limited employment opportunities outside of teaching, domestic and secretarial work. Most of the women who emigrated did so as soon as they finished secondary school. Although some of the women described their class status as 'comfortable' or 'well-off' by today's standards, many of those who were able to migrate were from the better-off class. Young British women who were considering career options during the post-war period were faced with a number of opportunities. Upon finishing secondary school at age fourteen, they possessed the necessary skills to access plentiful employment in the burgeoning clerical fields, light factory work and re-tail sales positions, but they required further training to enter a skilled occupation. Although the reasons for working provided by both the Caribbean and British women in the oral interviews defies easy generalizations, the dominant reason for many was the pursuit of a career. In the words of one interviewee, 'I could make better of myself'.[7] For Caribbean women that necessarily meant going overseas.

Jeanette P. left Antigua at the age of eighteen to begin her training as a nurse in 1958, later taking a certificate in midwifery. She did the first part of her training in the West Middlesex Hospital, London, and the second part in Kirkcaldy, Scotland. Commenting on her arrival in Scotland, Jeanette stated:

> I couldn't understand a word they said when I went there first, and the fun-niest thing, of all the midwives, none was Scottish and, again, I was the only West Indian, only black person; the rest were Irish, and a few English.[8]

Young women who chose nursing as a career were influenced by their cul-ture, religion and early socialization. The universal characterization of women as naturally and innately 'healing', 'caring' and 'nurturing' melds perfectly with the image of the nurse, one influenced thoroughly by nineteenth-century, upper-class notions of the 'best' of female attributes. Women were exhorted to these ideas in church and schools, and within the household all domestic duties were custom-arily undertaken by women. In addition, altruistic notions of caring for others, inspired in some by Christian belief, informed their decision to enter nursing. Statements such as 'I've always wanted to be a nurse and care for others' were reiterated throughout the interviews.[9] Some had family members who were nurses and spoke highly of the occupation.[10]

The development of professional nursing was influenced by a class-based professional ethic that saw the promotion of traditionally female occupations, including teaching and social work. By depicting good nursing skills as first and foremost inherent in women by virtue of their greater capacity for compassion, and then by fostering the ideals of good character and responsibility, the image of nurses as upstanding, respectable members of the community emerged.[11] One British midwife stated that when she was about the district in her uniform, there was no area in Aberdeen, Scotland, to which she was afraid, or unable, to go. Her profession was a source of protection.[12] A young woman considering a career in nursing could be assured, along with her parents, that the field she was entering would not sully her reputation in any way. In fact, her social status might be enhanced.

Despite the competition from other occupations, particularly those with fewer restrictions on a worker's time and how it was spent, nursing did not lose the cachet it carried as a profession in the post-war period. It was one of the few occupations available to large numbers, upon attainment of a practical education of moderate duration and expense, that could provide status, fulfilment and reasonable wages. Some Caribbean women were in the position to benefit from academic scholarships available to Commonwealth students who were unable to meet the financial requirements for their education.

In 1949, for example, at the age of seventeen, Vera C. left Trinidad for England on a government scholarship. She applied to the nursing programme because 'they [England] needed nurses'. It took Vera five years to complete her training, four years for her nursing diploma with another year for midwifery certification. She remained an extra year in Britain but returned to Trinidad upon completion of her training in accordance with the stipulations of the scholarship regulations.[13]

Nurse training was offered in Britain through hospital schools with strict residency requirements. Hospitals were provided with a source of inexpensive labour in the form of nursing students, who satisfied varying levels of care within an overworked National Health Service. Sheila F., a British nurse who entered training in 1946, stated that her first task as a student nurse was to sit and hold the hand of a dying man who was alone.[14] Before the end of her education, which spanned three years, a British-trained nurse would be expected to take on the responsibility for an entire ward during night shift. Many nurses who trained in Britain also undertook an additional year of training in midwifery, earning the necessary qualifications to deliver babies. In this study, eighteen of the twenty-two nurses were also midwives.

The student nurse was the backbone of nursing care for many institutions. The expenses of student life were offset by a number of allowances: uniforms were supplied by the hospital; a room was provided in the nurses' residence, with meals and laundry. Students were paid a modest stipend. The nurses themselves were responsible for shoes, stockings and underwear and any entertainment costs they incurred. As a bonus, local cinemas and theatres provided free passes to schools for the use of student nurses; and nurses were invited, en masse, to dances held in the community. Agnes B. remembered:

> In Glasgow in those days like your theatre or the cinemas, if they were having a trade show [movie] in the cinemas, they would send tickets into the Royal [Infirmary], the theatre usually sent free tickets for the afternoon performances. Like you got to a lot of things you didn't pay for them . . . if the police were having something or the army, the local barracks sometimes they sent in invitations for so many nurses to go . . .[15]

The remembrances of Caribbean nurse pupils were markedly different. Some nurses had first-hand experience of racism, whereas others learnt about it through their families, the media and other people's experiences. When Jean H. arrived in England, from Guyana, during the 1950s to begin her training as a nurse, she was surprised at the level of inequities meted out towards blacks 'because [racism] was not something I expected, but it was there'.[16] Nowhere was this truer than in respect to housing. Like most of her Caribbean counterparts who lived in residence, Jean escaped some of the blatant acts of racism experienced by others. Nevertheless, she pointed out:

I personally didn't experience that [racism] looking for room, because I didn't have to. But going with other people to look for accommodation, it was there. They would advertise room for rent: 'no coloureds'. Other times they advertised 'room for rent' or 'house for rent', and when you go and they see you are black, they would tell you its gone and close the door in your face. You would send a white person, they would accept them and say it was available.[17]

In one important aspect, entering nursing protected student nurses from having to find a place to live and being rejected because 'no coloureds are allowed'.

THE MIGRATION OF CARIBBEAN WOMEN

Jean's presence in England as a participant in the racially charged atmosphere of the 1950s and 1960s was integrally related to the broader processes of uneven development within the Caribbean periphery and the world capitalist system. Although investments in the Caribbean during the 1950s and 1960s created what some scholars characterize as a 'boom period', the majority of the people did not share in the prosperity of the national income; there was high unemployment in most Caribbean regions. Subsequently, a large number of Caribbean people were forced to migrate, seeking markets where they could sell their labour power. Thus, Caribbean peoples began the mass migration to Britain in search of opportunities for well-paid jobs in an industrialized nation. They chose Britain not least because they had retained the legal right to enter, settle and work there.[18] Efforts to resolve the labour shortage in certain sectors of the economy of post-war Britain produced changes to existing exclusionary policies. None of these processes, though, implied immediate acceptance of the Caribbean communities.

Migrating to Britain was difficult for some of the Caribbean young women. Their expectations of Britain, buttressed by a 'narrative of the nation',[19] which circulated in the Caribbean, led to feelings of disengagement and loneliness. After twenty-one days at sea, Dorothy J., only seventeen at the time, waited with anticipation for her brother to pick her up in Southampton. Dorothy poignantly relates her first reaction to Britain:

The first thing I noticed were the houses, I thought that going to England would have been like the fairy tales, the nursery rhymes right from the books. I thought you'll see castles, and it wasn't like that. I knew I wouldn't find the streets paved with gold, but the houses, well, my heart sank and I thought, 'that's England'. It was also May or June but it was still cold, and I was cold; it wasn't what I expected.[20]

In Britain, young women from the Caribbean who went to train as nurses learned for the first time that blackness was symbolic and had meaning – one that was not always positive in mainstream Britain. For Dorothy, race, coupled with gender and age, played a role in terms of how she was treated by her peers. Being the youngest nurse, she noticed that even though it was standard practice to use the title 'nurse' along with the first name, her mostly white colleagues ignored this practice when they referred to her. It was not until the British head nurse overheard the probationers and openly chastised them that they used the appropriate title.[21] Black nursing students and nurses also had to deal with overt forms of racism, expressed by patients, nurses, hospital kitchen staff and cleaners. Dorothy related the following incident:

> I remember this one woman said to me, 'is it true that black people live in trees?' I used to think these people were so stupid. I used to say 'these white people come to the West Indies and preach Christianity and all sort of things to us, and when you go to their country, you find out that they're the stupid ones because of the things they would ask and what they could come up with.' You'd wonder how could these people think about some things you wouldn't think about.[22]

Dorothy ignored the possibility that some statements had been intentionally provocative. She continued:

> And they really thought we were monkeys, and they'll talk to you on the floor, but once they got off the floor [off duty], they didn't bother with you. But then most of the black nurses knew that's what it was and they cared for themselves . . . they keep to themselves. At least that's what I did, some of the other black nurses mixed with and had friends, white friends, that they were close to and would go out with.[23]

Dorothy's experience of racism while working and training in Britain was definitely not an isolated experience; it was indicative of Caribbean nurses' experiences. However, the nurses did not allow themselves to be victimized by racism and they maintained their sanity by developing survival strategies to deal with the forms of discrimination. Black nurses socialized with their white counterparts when they felt accepted and comfortable; the alternatives were to limit social relations to other Caribbean immigrants or to keep to themselves. The reality of outsider status, marked by state repression, lack of upward mobility in many occupations, and inadequate housing in post-war Britain,[24] therefore, touched immigrant nurses directly. They experienced racism, and they knew it.

CARIBBEAN AND BRITISH NURSE MIGRATION TO CANADA

Why did both sets of interviewees, the British-born and most Caribbean-born nurses, emigrate to Canada shortly after the completion of their training? Both groups of women stated that they saw migration as an opportunity for escape, and a gateway to dignified middle-class employment within a prosperous economy. Many commented upon a feeling of dissatisfaction with some aspect of their lives in the UK.

The pursuit of new experiences propelled these, and others, across the Atlantic. One British nurse saw her position at the Hamilton General Hospital in Ontario as temporary, as a stopover on her way around the world.[25] Others had given themselves time limits, the most common being two years, to settle in and make a decision to either stay or to continue the quest.[26] Even though the opportunity presented itself for her to stay in England, Jennette P. refused and went to Antigua. The island was not the same as she remembered; but returning to England was not an alternative. Job postings in English magazines indicated that there were nursing jobs available in Canada. She remembered:

> I looked them up and found a hospital, I didn't even know there was a London, Ontario till I looked it up and found this hospital looking for nurses, and I wrote and got offered the job. They told me to write immigration and I wrote them.[27]

Others recalled hearing of the nursing shortage and migrated because of the wage opportunities; other nurses were encouraged to emigrate because they had family members who were already in Canada. Thus, migration was not driven by a single goal of earning a better salary. One nurse stated simply: 'it seemed like the right thing to do'.[28] Whether emigrating directly from the Caribbean or initially to Britain and then to Canada, Caribbean nurses encountered challenges that continued to shape their consciousness.

Large numbers of black colonial immigrants arrived in Britain immediately after the Second World War; however, in Canada, racist exclusionary policies during the 1940s and 1950s prevented such large numbers of black people from immigrating and promoted the immigration of British subjects, including trained nurses.[29] This movement was favoured and assisted in all possible ways. Immigration from the Caribbean was essentially closed until the redrafting of the Canadian Immigration Act to incorporate the points system in 1967; this allowed the admission of immigrants based on certain labour and skill requirements. Prior to this, because of their professional status and the need for nurses, the state permitted a limited number of Caribbean nurses to train and/or work in Canada as 'cases of exceptional merit'.[30] These women were viewed as exceptional by the state – as the group that would help white Canadians adjust to the presence of blacks in Canada. With the emergence of a more 'liberal' and 'non-discriminatory' points system in 1967, the immigration of Caribbean people reached its historical height during the 1970s and 1980s.[31]

THE SHORTAGE IN CANADA

The emigration of Caribbean and British nurses to Canada was in direct response to the pressing need for nursing services arising out of the transformation of the post-war Canadian economy. The National Employment Service, in its annual report, *Supply and Demand of University Graduates*, urged employment and guidance counsellors to encourage young women to pursue a nursing career.[32] As more and more Canadian women entered into employment that had been traditionally unavailable to them, for many, teaching and nursing were no longer their first occupational option. With the assistance of the federal government, a range of endeavours were undertaken to increase the number of nurses in the provinces. Funds were allotted to provide bursaries to high-school girls to stimulate interest in nursing as a career. Recommendations aimed at 'alleviating the manpower problem in nursing' included: subsidiary nursing programmes that required less training; a reduction in the turn-over rate; changing the unemployed status of over 25,000 nurses to employed; and increased immigration and reduced emigration.[33] However, when nursing associations spoke of increasing immigration they were not referring to immigrants from the Caribbean. They thought first of the UK or the USA, countries themselves facing shortages in nursing services. Immigrants from Scandinavia and the Ukraine were accepted into the country as nurses, although they were limited by language barriers and were expected to fill the lowest echelons of the nursing hierarchy. It was the failure of these initiatives to meet rising demand that led to the immigration of Caribbean nurses as the last alternative.

Unlike white nurses, who were admitted to Canada based on their general admissibility as immigrants, Caribbean nurses were admitted solely on their qualifications. Federal policies stipulated that the immigration of Caribbean nurses had to be authorized by an Order-in-Council, premised upon unambiguous evidence that applicants were ready for registration and had already found suitable employment with a hospital that was aware of their race.[34] As in Britain, there was concern that black immigration could threaten the moral or social fabric of the nation. Caribbean nurses were perhaps unaware of the racist climate to which they were immigrating. Although restrictive immigration policies limited the immigration of Caribbean nurses directly from the Caribbean, there was no indication from the nurses themselves or other sources that immigration officials were interested in limiting the migration of British-trained Caribbean nurses. The fact that British-trained Caribbean nurses were disproportionately represented in the larger study suggests that it was easier for them to immigrate than their Caribbean-trained counterparts.

Nurses employed in the UK were well aware of the nursing shortage in Canada. Canadian hospitals sent recruitment agents to Britain, who toured the regions in search of nurses to bring back to their institutions. Six of the nurses in our research came to Canada that way: three black, three white. Hospitals in Canada promised better pay, as well as vacation, location and vocation inducements. Seventeen of the nurses who emigrated did so as single women. The nurses recorded a certain amount of satisfaction in the fact that they were sought after for their skills. Susan G., a British midwife, commented: 'it was so nice to feel wanted'.[35] Hospitals offered assisted passages to facilitate recruitment, although none in our study took advantage of these terms. It emerged as a point of pride that they paid their own way, even if it meant borrowing money from family members. Assisted passages did not always work to the advantage of the nurse. Some immigrant nurses had to stay in situations that were intolerable because they could not leave the employ of the hospital until their passage had been repaid. During one particular episode of hostility between Maureen J., a newly arrived British nurse, and a Canadian nurse, a statement was thrown at Maureen to the effect that she had to do what the Canadian said; she could not go anywhere until her passage was repaid. Maureen spat back that she wasn't in debt to the hospital and she didn't have to stay if she didn't want to. This response silenced the Canadian nurse. Maureen shared this incident at the time not only with her fellow immigrant nurses but also with the Director of Nursing. The Canadian nurse received a reprimand and Maureen received an apology. This was joyfully seen as a victory for all the immigrant nurses at the hospital.[36] Interestingly, none of the Caribbean nurses recruited in Britain referred to the possibility of assisted passages. Was that not an option? Were they, perhaps, too marginal?

WORKING IN CANADA

Many of the nurses who migrated to Canada encountered Canada for the first time through their dealings with a hospital administrator or their representative visiting the UK on a recruitment drive. In the marketplace of hospital nursing, the shortage of nurses was so acute that regular hiring procedures could be bypassed in favour of expedient measures. This was true in the case of Agnes B., a midwife, who was unable to keep her interview appointment due to an unexpected delivery. As the interviewer could not reschedule the meeting, a friend, who was also being interviewed, spoke on her behalf. After a brief telephone conversation, Agnes found herself with a position in southern Ontario at the Hamilton General Hospital.[37] All the nurses interviewed commented favourably on the hospital administrator and representative who they met during the recruitment drives. For those who arrived with jobs arranged through the mail, their reception at their respective hospitals was also remembered as warm and friendly. The Director of Nursing was eager to see them settled and comfortable in their accommodation, usually in the hospital nurses residence.[38]

Adjustment is a major theme in the history of the profession and the history of immigration. Many nurses interviewed remarked on the differences in the work environments between Canada and the UK. Invariably, the British nurses found Canadian hospitals to be more relaxed in atmosphere, less rigid and authoritarian. They saw this as a welcome change from working in British hospitals ruled – in their memories – by an iron-fisted matron and where the ward sister struck terror into the staff nurse, and the staff nurse into the student. One British nurse commented: '. . . there were some witches, believe me. You haven't met a British Ward Sister, you haven't lived. They ruled the roost'.[39] It was felt that the first thing a nurse learned in Britain was the hierarchy and her place within it. The same nurse continued:

> [you] were the lowest of the low, you're probbies, probationers, and everybody sort of looks down on you . . . when you went to a ward then you'd found out that you'd be the lowest one and then you had to quickly decide or find

out who was next . . . every three months there's a new class come in . . . so somebody's three months ahead of you but they're still in the same year as you so they're the ones you can go to. You can't go to someone in their second year . . . there was still a lot of that went on long after I finished training and you didn't get too friendly with the ward sister.[40]

The student's circle of acquaintances was limited to those who occupied the same place in the hierarchy, regardless of class, and, unless initiated from above, that was as far as her sphere extended. Albeit modified and lessened, this continued after graduation and entrance into a hospital post. In Canada, the Caribbean and British nurses experienced a different situation. Although still within a hierarchy, they felt that those occupying the most senior positions were approachable. One nurse who had been having difficulties with a Canadian nurse felt a sense of trepidation when she was asked to tell her side to the Director of Nursing. The Director then spoke with the Canadian nurse and hostilities ended. The interest shown by the Director in the problems encountered on the floor was viewed in a highly positive manner, and accelerated the acclimatization process. The nurse in question felt that this type of personal involvement had been missing in British hospitals.[41] Nonetheless, although some of the senior nurses might have taken a more personal interest in their staff, there were still barriers between levels of nursing service. One British nurse recalled that during her first communal dining experience in the hospital residence, after listening to one Canadian nurse, 'go on at great lengths about how different things were in Canada, no class divisions and such and how everybody was equal no matter how much money your father had', she proceeded to take a seat along with her friend, another newly arrived British nurse, at a table along one wall. In a very short time she was politely, but firmly, tapped on her shoulder and told that only head nurses sat at that table. 'So much for equality' she commented sardonically.[42]

The British-trained Caribbean nurses, on the other hand, appeared not to have minded or disliked the rigidity of the British hospital system. The challenge for them in Canada was credentials, and in this singled-minded pursuit they emphasized the value and standards of the British hospitals. Myrna B., a Caribbean nurse, refused to complete additional courses to receive her registration because, according to Myrna, she 'had learned everything in England, there was nothing more for me to learn'.[43]

Although both the Caribbean and British nurses entered Canada as fully trained nurses, they entered the healthcare system as nurse assistants. Despite having one qualification extraordinary in the Canadian context (midwifery certification), many nurses had to take written exams for licensure, most often in obstetrics and paediatrics; this was viewed by all as absurd. However, with their midwifery certificates ignored, the relative lack of obstetrics training in their nursing education became a liability that required them to complete the necessary course and sit the exam. Nurse assistants were paid at a lower rate and performed many of the less-skilled, less palatable, aspects of nursing care. For example, Caribbean nurse Elaine E., a state enrolled nurse, immigrated to Canada in 1969. Elaine worked as a non-registered nursing assistant due to the difficulties that administrative bodies introduced when interpreting British qualifications in a Canadian context. Both Elaine and Myrna felt, however, that their British-trained skills and experience made them more qualified than their Canadian counterparts.[44] Nevertheless, they were relegated to work as subsidiary workers. According to Elaine, 'I was more qualified to be doing more than what I was doing, but I was not, as far as it was established in Canada'. She claimed that as a non-registered nursing assistant, she was responsible for what she classified as 'non-educational tasks'. Elaine blamed the College of Nurses for overlooking her qualifications: 'they didn't think it was up to their standard . . . having done two years [in England] when theirs [in Canada] is just a ten-month programme'.[45] For many of the nurses, their time as assistants was limited because they fulfilled the requirements by sitting the necessary exams; some had to sit them a few times. This failure to pass on first attempt they attributed to the difference in examination methods. Nursing exams in the UK were essay answers in response to questions; in Canada the exams were multiple choice, a format alien to the British-trained nurses.

PRACTICE RESTRICTIONS

Many midwives had difficulties adjusting to the skill restrictions they now faced practising in Canada. This emerged as a major issue of re-adjustment and an alienating experience. Upon their employment in Canada, the nurses who held midwifery certificates were instructed that they were not allowed to deliver babies. One nurse said that her supervisor informed her that 'under no condition, absolutely none, was I to deliver a baby. But babies, who tells them when to come? But better a fireman or a taxi driver than me'. After months of working on the obstetrical ward of a Hamilton hospital, this nurse transferred to the maternity ward. She had felt cheated, after labouring for hours alongside the mother, to be deprived of the joy of helping the baby in the final stage of her journey. That part was taken over by the doctor, who conveniently arrived just in time.[46]

The former midwives were limited not only in the physical practice of delivering babies. They were also not allowed to present a medical opinion to the expectant mothers, even when expressly asked. In all cases they were to defer to the doctor in charge, regardless of whether they agreed with the advice. One British nurse, a former midwife, relates an instance where an expectant mother, anxious over her baby's lack of movement, pleaded with the nurse to tell her what she thought:

> I went in and I said look, no matter what I tell you I'm not allowed to tell you anything, no matter what I find I can't tell you. I said it's forbidden in this country and the mother said – I'm a Scot – will you pretend you're in Scotland and tell me what's wrong. It won't get out of this room. So I examined her, told her what I thought . . . one doctor said her baby was alive another had said her baby was dead. I said I'm not a doctor, so what I'm telling you . . . is not a doctor's opinion. I can't go quoted . . . so I told her

. . . Back home I could've sat with her, talked to her about it; that would have been acceptable.[47]

A trained midwife, Sandra W., immigrated to Canada in 1971. She highlighted her own experience as a pregnant mother to illustrate a number of points ranging from the lack of information given to pregnant mothers in Canada, to how limited general nurse training was in Canada with respect to childbirth, and how doctors dominated obstetrics. Sandra remembered:

When I was pregnant, no one told me anything. I didn't tell them that I was a nurse. I didn't go to the doctor until I was 6 months. I knew I was having a good pregnancy, no complications. I had the child and still no one told me what to do. If I were a new mother, I wouldn't know what to do.[48]

She explicated the difference between the doctor's role in childbirth in England and Canada:

Over here, [Canada] most of the doctors do the delivery. I took that to mean that the nurses really had nothing to do in terms of examining the baby. In England when you do midwifery, you have to know everything about labour. The nurse is there, even if it's a student nurse [she] examines you. You were told everything about the pregnancy and what to look for. You don't have to be a midwife to know that.[49]

According to Sandra, student nurses in Britain were expected to check for abnormalities once a pregnant patient entered the hospital, a procedure that was absent in Canada. Getting acquainted and accustomed to the Canadian system would have been a challenge for Sandra, had she not been employed in a hospital with a number of British-trained nurses. The presence of sizeable numbers of these nurses within the Canadian healthcare system eased the transition of their integration into Canada.

Lilli Johnson, who is currently retired, enjoyed an extensive career in England and Scotland as a midwife before migrating to Canada in 1960. Similar to her counterparts discussed in this chapter thus far, Johnson too renounced the way in which patriarchy structures the gender and racial division of labour, and the relationship between doctors and nurses. She explains:

They give you no responsibility. The doctor has to order everything. Although it seems to be getting better, it seems all they [doctors] want is a 'handmaiden'. There are so many British-trained nurses who have their midwifery training, but none of them are accredited for it here.[50]

Instead of working on a ward where she must watch doctors deliver babies, Lilli chose to pursue additional studies that would enable her to work as a public health nurse. Her criticisms regarding the authority doctors have in the birthing process demonstrates a keen understanding of how gender informs the relationship between doctors and nurses.

In many other ways the nursing skills of the migrant nurses were curtailed. They could not remove dressings or sutures unless expressly told to and, in many cases they did so, albeit supervised by the attending physician.[51] They could not administer simple pain relief unless the doctor had ordered it on the chart. Moira B., a British nurse, had taken it upon herself to give an aspirin to a patient with a headache. She was called to task, asked to explain herself and was told to sign a form acknowledging her error. She refused to do so, insistent that she had done no wrong. In the end, a doctor, one who was familiar with British nursing practices, covered for her by ordering aspirin on the chart.[52]

Elaine and other Caribbean nurses complained of deskilling when they migrated to Canada, relegated as they were to the bottom of the nursing hierarchy.[53] Myrna pointed out that her nursing experience in England was incomparable to her nursing experience in Canada. According to Myrna, 'nursing in England, you were a nurse, you were taught everything, whereas here [in Canada] you learn some things'.[54] In the UK, these nurses had been trained to take the initiative in such care-giving matters as changing dressings, removing sutures, utilizing common remedies such as poultices and plasters, and in dispensing certain kinds of pharmaceuticals, such as aspirin. Doctors held the prescription licence, but they worked closely with nurses to provide the information needed for them to make an informed decision. One British nurse said that they 'had a much better relationship with doctors in Scotland, especially if you were the ward sister . . . they relied on you so much and accepted you as a fellow sort of professional . . . maybe not quite an equal but almost an equal'.[55] For these nurses, effective nursing meant being able to demonstrate in practice what they had been taught as students. This sense of alienation – extending back decades – was ever present in the oral interviews. These nurses, black and white, had been deskilled. That grievance crossed the colour barrier. Indeed, it obliterated, for the moment, the colour barrier. Speaking individually to different interviewees, the message was the same: we could have done – we should have been permitted to do – so much more. This is a phenomenon of British-trained nurses in post-war Canada. In this one respect, race or geographic origin was tempered as opposed to immaterial.

Structural changes in the occupation during this period also affected how Caribbean and British immigrant nurses understood and explained their responsibilities within nursing. With the introduction of subsidiary education programmes, bedside care in Canada was no longer the purview of Registered Nurses, but of nursing assistants. Once the immigrant nurses completed Canadian licensing requirements, therefore, they found contact with patients curtailed within the Canadian hospital model. The British-trained nurses, however, had difficulties with the allocation of duties that did not include adequate bedside care, which they had been taught in the UK was a fundamental nursing role. Vera C. stated:

We had [in Britain] to spend time with the patients and that meant a lot, psychologically, it was very good medicine. Our whole training, when it was

given to us, we understood that it was very personal – that type of psychological treatment was good for patients – sometimes they needed that more than
the medicine.[56]

It is apparent from the evidence that the British-trained nurses had absorbed
a nursing ideal, now judged in the Canadian context of rapid expansion to be
expensive and outdated. It is of interest that the immigrant nurses' concern for
their status within the profession was pursued within their conception of the profession: the increased status of the nurse *vis-à-vis* the nursing assistant worked to
their long-term advantage, but it failed to meet the ideals of the profession as they
had learned them.

The constraints on the time available for the provision of bedside care in the
Canadian system affected their sense of identity as nurses. This is significant; for
many of these women, as they recalled, the reason they chose nursing was their
desire to 'care for others'. Pat, a British nurse, recalled her first day on a Canadian
ward. The Canadian nurse assigned to work with her refused to show her around
or to help her in any way. She had said to Pat: 'I've got enough of my own to do.
I haven't got time to show you what to do . . . That's your side of the hallway and
that's mine'.[57] This structure of ward work in Canada contributed to a sense of
isolation among the nurses. Instead of pairing up and working together as they
'panned and bathed and made the beds', as in Britain, in Canada they worked
separately, one on each side of the ward. Similarly, the division in care services
was perceived to pit one ward against another, particularly in maternity hospitals,
where labour and delivery was separate from maternity, which was separate from
the nursery. It was not the care of mother and child combined, but of 'mother'
and 'child' separately. This process of specialization was viewed as a retrograde
step. [58]

CONCLUSION

It is the experience of being in the UK during training, when occupational identity was formed, that pulled the reminiscences of Caribbean and British nurses
towards common ground regarding issues of workplace autonomy, the process
of deskilling and professional pride. And whereas race and cultural difference are
never absent from the world of work, the women interviewed respond primarily
as nurses to the questions about their experiences about work. However, as their
experiences indicate, this common ground was shaded by tones of racism and cultural disunity. For Caribbean nurses, racism was more blatant in Britain, although
their experience of it was clouded by their own segregation within residential
nursing schools and away from the larger British society. In Canada at this time,
racism was not as apparent, although in hindsight the lack of a language or the
ability to speak about racism contributed to muting its presence both within the
profession and within the hospital. Vera T. stated:

The issue of racism was not evident and apparent at that time as it is now.
There were so few of us here that they [whites] had not begun to panic, to

feel afraid or intimidated by our presence . . . on the other hand in the hospital we were a minority and we were just concerned with doing our work. They [hospital administrators] seemed to want us more than anything.[59]

For British nurses, despite the racial similarities between Canada and the United Kingdom, cultural disunity served to alienate British nurses from their Canadian counterparts and, indeed, many of the British nurses expressed affinity with the other immigrant groups arriving in Canada during this time. One nurse referred to the post-war Canadian milieu as 'the united nations' in reference to the myriad nationalities found among the newly arrived immigrants;[60] and, in fact, ten of the British nurses married non-Canadian men. The experiences of these nurses provide insight into the problems and rewards faced by immigrant workers upon arrival in a new country. Despite the difficulties they encountered, the majority of both Caribbean and white British nurses expressed satisfaction with their decision to remain in Canada, if not in nursing. Deskilling and practice restrictions were a fact of life for British-trained nurses in Canada. Both British and Caribbean nurses experienced similar restrictions, which they attributed to differences in nurse training and practice expectations rather than attempts at racial or cultural discrimination, whether overt or covert. Their identity as British-trained nurses served to mediate their experiences of racial and cultural disunity within the dominant Canadian culture. For Caribbean nurses, the superiority in which they held their British training affected their experiences of racial discrimination. They were not alone in this; British nurses also felt alienated within the work environment due to practice restrictions. Both groups experienced occupational dissatisfaction, to varying degrees. Caribbean and British nurses found themselves in similar situations and practice circumstances, further solidifying their bond as British-trained nurses. It was not until the later 1970s that focused attention on Canadian multiculturalism contributed to the creation of an understanding of racism that gave a clearer meaning to, and a language that could express, the discriminatory practices of the past. These women had a vested interest in being accepted as professionals in the Canadian system, and their continued insistence that the British system is superior is a response to their marginalization. It is a testament to the success of the British nurse training process that it resulted in the cohesion of an occupational identity that crossed racial lines, and served to support nurses in the face of occupational and racial discrimination.

NOTES

1   Both authors wish to thank the Hannah Institute for the History of Medicine for their support in funding this research with a History of Medicine Studentship, held by Margaret Shkimba in summer 1995 and a History of Medicine Doctoral Scholarship held by Karen Flynn 1999–2000. The tapes are in the possession of the interviewers. Pseudonyms are used throughout.
2   Agnes B., interview by Margaret Shkimba, tape recording, Hamilton, Ontario, August, 1995.
3   'Recruitment and training of nurses in Great Britain', *Ministry of Labour Gazette*, 1947, Vol. 55, pp. 336–7.

4   B. Ladoucer and P. Spence (eds), *Blackouts to Bright Lights: Canadian War Bride Stories*, Vancouver: Ronsdale Press, 1995; B. Wicks, *Promise You'll Take Care of my Daughter: the Remarkable War Brides of World War II*, Toronto: Stoddart Press, 1992; P. O'Hara (ed.), *From Romance to Reality*, Cobalt, Ontario: Highway Book Shop, 1983.

5   M. Silvera, *Silenced: Talks with Working Class Caribbean Women About their Lives and Struggles as Domestic Workers in Canada*, Toronto: Sister Vision Press, 1983; P. Daenzer, *Regulating Class Privilege: Immigrant Servants in Canada, 1940–1990*, Toronto: Canadian Scholars Press, 1993; S. Arat-Koc, 'In the privacy of our own home: foreign domestic workers as a solution to the crisis of the domestic sphere in Canada', *Studies in Political Economy* 1989, Vol. 28, pp. 33–58; A. Calliste, 'Canada's immigration policy and domestics from the Caribbean: The second domestic scheme', in J. Vorst (ed.), *Race, Class, Gender: Bonds and Barriers* 2nd edn, Toronto: Garamond Press, 1991, pp. 136–68; V. Satzewich, 'Racism and Canadian immigration policy: The government's view of Caribbean migration', *Canadian Ethnic Studies,* 1989, Vol. 21, (1), pp. 77–97; J. A. Schultz, 'White man's country: Canada and the West Indian immigrant, 1900–1965', *American Review of Canadian Studies,* 1982, Vol. 12 (1), pp. 53–64.

6   Canada. *Canada Year Book*, 1962.

7   Dorothy J., interview by Karen Flynn, tape recording, Rexdale, Ontario, 29 February 2000.

8   Jeanette P., interview by Karen Flynn, tape recording, North York, Ontario, 8 October 1999.

9   Lilli J., interview by Karen Flynn, tape recording, Scarborough, Ontario, 9 August 1999; Theresa T., interview by Margaret Shkimba, tape recording, Hamilton, Ontario, August 1995.

10   Sandra W., interview by Karen Flynn, tape recording, Toronto, Ontario, 5 January 2000; Agnes B. 'August, 1995'.

11   P. O. Jardine, 'An urban middle-class calling: women and the emergence of modern nursing education at the Toronto General Hospital 1881–1914', *Urban History Review/Revue d'histoire urbaine*, 1989, Vol. XVII, (3), pp. 177–90.

12   Sheila F., interview by Margaret Shkimba, tape recording, Hamilton, Ontario, August 1995.

13   Vera C., interview by Karen Flynn, tape recording, Rexdale, Ontario, 5 January 1995.

14   Sheila F., August 1995.

15   Agnes B., August 1995.

16   Dorothy J., February 2000.

17   Jean H., interview by Karen Flynn, tape recording, Scarborough, Ontario, 8 August.

18   J. Solomos, *Race and Racism in Britain,* New York: St Martin's Press, 1993.

19   'Narrative of the nation' refers to the memories, myths and symbols used to construct and support the idea of nation throughout the empire. See: H. Bahbha, *Nation and Narration*, New York: Routledge, 1994.

20   Dorothy J., February 2000.

21   Ibid.

22   Ibid.

23   Ibid.

24   B. Carter, C. Harris, and S. Joshi, 'The 1951–55 Conservative government and the racialization of black migration', in K. Owsu (ed.), *Black British Culture and Society: a Text Reader*, London: Routledge, 2000.

25   Vera T., interview by Margaret Shkimba, tape recording, Hamilton, Ontario, August 1995.

26   Mary W., interview by Margaret Shkimba, tape recording, Hamilton, Ontario, August 1995.

27   Jeanette P., October 1999.
28   Lilli J., August 1999.
29   B. Singh Bolaria and P. S. Li, *Racial Oppression in Canada*, Toronto: Garamond Press, 1988; Solomos, *Race and Racism*.
30   Agnes Calliste, ' "Women of exceptional merit": immigration of Caribbean nurses to Canada', *Canadian Journal of Women and the Law/Revue juridique La femme et le droit*, 1993, Vol. 6, pp. 85–102.
31   L. M. Jakubowski, *Immigration and the Legalization of Racism*, Halifax, Nova Scotia: Fernwood Press, 1997.
32   Canada. National Employment Service. *Supply and Demand of University Graduates*, 1954–1959.
33   Ontario Public Archives, RG10 Health Records, letter to the Premier from Christine Livingstone, President, Registered Nursing Association of Ontario, 21 January 1957, RG10–106–92–1.
34   Calliste, 'Women of exceptional merit'.
35   Susan G., interview by Margaret Shkimba, tape recording, Hamilton, Ontario, August 1995.
36   Maureen J., interview by Margaret Shkimba, tape recording, Hamilton, Ontario, August 1995.
37   Agnes B., August 1995.
38   Susan G., August 1995; Sheila F., August 1995.
39   Vera T., August 1995.
40   Ibid.
41   Mary W., August 1995.
42   Maureen J., August 1995.
43   Myrna B, interview by Karen Flynn, tape recording, Brampton, Ontario, 29 May 1995. K. Flynn, 'Experience and identity: Black immigrant nurses in Canada, 1950–1980', in M. Epp, F. Iacovetta and F. Swyripa (eds), *Sisters or Strangers: Immigrant, Ethnic and Racialised Women in Canadian History*, Toronto; University of Toronto Press, 2004, pp. 381–98.
44   Myrna B., ibid.; Elaine E, interview by Karen Flynn, tape recording, Markham, Ontario, May 1995. K. Flynn, 'Proletarianization, Professionalization and Caribbean Immigrant Nurses', *Canadian Women's Studies Journal*, 1998, Vol. 18, pp. 57–64.
45   Elaine E., May 1995.
46   Vera T., August 1995.
47   Maureen J., August 1995.
48   Sandra W., January 2000. K. Flynn, *Sisters or Strangers*, p. 389.
49   Ibid.
50   Lilli J., interview by Karen Flynn, tape recording, Scarborough, Ontario, August 1999.
51   Vera T., August 1995.
52   Moira B., interview by Margaret Shkimba, tape recording, August, 1995.
53   Elaine E., May 1995.
54   Myrna B., May 1995.
55   Agnes B., August 1995.
56   Vera T., August 1995. K. Flynn, 'Proletarianization and Professionalization', p. 58.
57   Pat K., interview by Margaret Shkimba, tape recording, August 1995.
58   Agnes B., August 1995.
59   Vera T., August 1995.
60   Agnes B., August 1995.

10 'Beware of worthless imitations'

Advertising in nursing periodicals, c. 1888–1945

Elaine Thomson

Advertisements are one of the most influential means of communication in the modern Western economy. Since the Victorian period, print media advertising has evolved from simple line drawings and fulsome accounts of product attributes into sophisticated visual constructions involving the persuasive use of images and words that shape and reflect our aspirations, our self-image and our perceptions of others. As an influential form of modern media, advertisements have attracted the critical attention of scholars from diverse disciplinary backgrounds, including sociology and gender studies,[1] linguistics and semiotics,[2] history and art history,[3] as well as drawing critical scrutiny from marketers and advertisers themselves.[4]

Even without these scholarly accounts we, as consumers, have become increasingly critical of advertisements. In the twenty-first century, when the average individual living in the developed world sees or hears about 500 commercial messages a day,[5] we consider ourselves to be streetwise about advertising and the moneymaking objectives of the advertisers and marketers who create it. Even as we buy a new product, we can acknowledge that advertisements are manipulative, that they try to sell us things we neither need nor want through the use of cleverly engineered images – images that show an idealized social reality to which we can only aspire. Attaining this ideal, of course – so promotional material encourages us to believe – can be achieved only by purchasing the goods or services advertised.[6] As Judith Williamson observed, one of the reasons why modern advertisements are so persuasive is because they do not simply sell us a product or a consumer good. Rather, in providing us with a structure of meaning for products and commodities, a language of objects that translates into a language of people, advertisements are 'selling us something besides consumer goods . . . they are selling us ourselves'.[7]

Implicit in Williamson's structuralist–semiotic interpretation is the notion of ideology: the understanding that advertisements are inherently based on a culturally determined misrecognition of the real relationship between certain ideas, for example the status of nature and culture and, in the context of this paper, the notion that women are naturally fitted to be nurses and that nurses themselves 'are who and what they are because that is who and what they should be'.[8]

But how have the nurse and her profession fared at the hands of advertisers? The portrayal of women in advertisements has been a subject of outrage among feminists since the 1970s,[9] but have images aimed at professional women been similarly ideologically charged? The image of the nurse has received a certain amount of scholarly attention.[10] Apart from Julia Hallam's study of professional boundaries and media image, however, the importance of advertising in the construction and maintenance of roles and stereotypes within nursing has been sadly overlooked by historians.[11] Yet advertisements are central to modern consumer culture. Indeed, they themselves are carriers of culture. By necessity they employ words and images that resonate with, and appeal to, the target audience. Without providing an identifiable visual link between the consumer and the object to be consumed, their impact would be minimal. In this way, advertisements aimed at nurses form a discursive space where definitions of femininity, and of professional roles and identities, are endorsed and reproduced. They tell us much about the aspirations of the nurse, the way she was perceived – by herself and others – and her place in medicine and in society.[12] Furthermore, advertisements form a site that links, and draws attention to, technological and social change within the medical and nursing professions.[13] Indeed, the language and images of advertising also reveal social and political changes within society at large, as well as indicating more immediate changes in the patterns of consumption among their target market.[14]

Clearly, advertisements hold much of interest for the historian of nursing. Focusing on the period from *c.* 1888 to *c.* 1945 this chapter will offer some preliminary explorations of this rich resource, charting its development from the use of simple line drawings to the emergence of the more sophisticated and persuasive techniques of the twentieth century. It will reveal the opportunities for advertisers presented by nursing periodicals, and indicate how wider social and political changes within society and within the profession of nursing are played out within the advertising pages of the nursing press. Finally, it will provide an opportunity to reflect on the way in which representations of the nurse in advertising, as a professional and as a consumer, changed and developed over time.

'IN TOUCH WITH MODERN METHODS': ADVERTISING IN THE NURSING PRESS TO *c.* 1900

The emergence of the periodical press was a distinctive feature of the development of print media in Victorian Britain. Periodicals were ideal vehicles for small advertisements, which could target a specific audience or class with particular interests. Almost simultaneous with these developments, following the Nightingale reforms of the 1860s and 1870s, nursing had emerged in Britain as a career for (usually single or widowed) middle-class women.[15] By the late Victorian period, nursing had developed a distinct professional ethos. Central to this was the appearance of national publications aimed specifically at this emergent group of educated, middle-class, working women, who possessed a disposable income and had distinctive consumer requirements. Periodicals such as *Nursing Mirror*, *Nursing Record* (both from 1888), *Nursing Notes* (from 1887) and the *Nurse's Journal* (from 1891) sprang up to meet the new and growing demand within the profession for news and information on nursing issues.

From the outset, nursing was perceived by its new recruits as a serious subject: one involving life and death, responsibility, commitment and extensive training. The editorial content of the new nursing journals mirrored these concerns, being serious in tone and content. Articles on nursing practice – such as bandaging techniques and the treatment of burns – the need for professional registration and new developments in medical and surgical procedures appeared alongside advertisements for uniforms and accessories, medical books and training courses, as well as employment opportunities in the voluntary hospitals, in public health, private nursing or teaching.[16] Throughout the period in question, therefore, nursing periodicals contained articles, and advertisements, which were of interest to nurses in all branches of the profession. It was to the private nurse, however, that the nursing press and the advertisements contained therein were of particular significance. At least half of those who completed their training in the late nineteenth and early twentieth centuries were destined to enter private nursing.[17] However, because of her isolation from the teaching hospitals, by the 1890s the private nurse was regarded as facing additional difficulties in staying 'in touch with modern methods'. To overcome this problem, commentators urged her to read 'at least one nursing paper carefully every week from cover to cover'. Not only would this keep her 'informed' about nursing methods, it would also allow her to stay abreast of the 'latest inventions', which could then be purchased for the patient.[18] The 'medical suppliers' she might need to patronize on behalf of her patient, for example, could best be located by reading the nursing press as 'all the best known of these advertise in the professional nursing journals.'[19] The private nurse was actively encouraged to 'make herself acquainted' with various brands and products – laxatives (Petrol-Agar or Agarol), maternity corsets (the Kestos Bust-Bodice), convalescent foods (Marmite or Bemax), for example – in order to 'advise the patient as to which is most suitable'. The perusal of advertisements, especially those that offered free samples on application to the manufacturer, was perceived as one of the best ways to do this.[20] From the very outset, therefore, with the private nurse exhorted to read nursing journals 'carefully every week from cover to cover' as a 'duty . . . to our professions and to ourselves',[21] these periodicals were afforded a wide, and interested, audience. As a result, nursing journals immediately attracted the attention of manufacturers and advertisers keen to get their products to as wide a market as possible.

Reflecting the seriousness of the life and commitments of the Victorian nurse, advertisements in this early period were made up of simple line drawings surmounted by endorsements for a product's efficacy and banners indicating the place where it could be bought and for what price.[22] Advertisements were factual in content and were generally concerned with promoting products that might be of use to the nurse – particularly the private nurse – in her professional capacity as carer of the sick and advisor of patients. The private nurse was required to 'carry with her a certain number of things,' at all times, including 'charts . . . scissors . . . catheters . . . dressing forceps'. In addition, she was called upon to advise her patient on the need to purchase other 'medical necessities . . . beds . . . bed pans, chairs, commodes . . . dressings,' and so on.[23] As a result, the nursing press abounded with advertisements for these and similar products. Bath chairs, bed pans, enema apparatus, 'diagnostic finger stalls, with aprons', as well as more inventive objects, such as the Relief Seat lavatory aid, the Noiseless Bucket or the Claxton Patented Ear Cap (for 'beautiful children disfigured by their prominent ears . . . Beware of worthless imitations') appeared consistently throughout the 1890s and into the first decade of the twentieth century.[24]

Advertisements for nurses' uniforms also made their appearance in the very first nursing journals.[25] Although the hospital nurse was required to purchase the uniform of her institution, the private nurse could wear 'whichever type she chooses' as long as it was 'well fitting, neat and spotlessly clean . . . A three weeks supply is advisable.'[26] The London-based firms Garrould's, Debenham and Freebody and Holdron's of Balham – the best-known manufacturers of nurses' uniforms – took out full-page advertisements to promote their stock of dresses, caps, capes, corsets and various accessories throughout the period in question.

Manufacturers of products that the private nurse, in her capacity as carer of the sick and convalescent, might use to revivify, sedate or purge their patients, appeared regularly. Franz Josef Natural Aperient Water advertised its 'dependable action' directly 'to nurses' as a laxative for the costive patient, for instance, whereas Van Houton's Cocoa was promoted as the ideal food for convalescents.[27] Not only were restoratives, sedatives and purgatives advertised for nurses to try on their patients, however, they were also advertised for the busy nurse to use herself. By the early twentieth century, advertisements were describing products as solutions to specific social and professional problems, rather than simply functional goods. An advertisement for '"Camp" the nurses' coffee' in 1907 exhorted the nurse to take a cup of this 'fresh [and] always delicious' product to stay awake and 'be ready for the night' (Figure 10.1).[28] In 1896 the Perfected Wyeth Beef Juice was given a full-page advertisement, claiming to be 'essential in the nervous exhaustion of sickness, convalescence, overwork and for the brain-fag of busy workers . . . Overworked nurses find it an invaluable pick-me-up'.[29]

From the 1890s advertisements for branded products appeared in nurses' periodicals. Products recognizable today, but with 'healthful' connotations, made some of their earliest public appearances in the pages of nursing magazines. Bovril and Oxo (both restoratives), Kellogg's (for bowel regularity), Nestlé (for babies) and Hovis (for bowels and digestion) were all given attributes to which the private nurse, as consumer on behalf of the invalid, nursing mother or constipated individual, could relate. Hovis bread and biscuits, for example, advertised using the usual litany of 'facts', appeared in *Nursing Notes* in 1893. It was 'recommended strongly by the medical profession; the only food that will prevent or cure indigestion [and] absolutely necessary for all growing children'.[30] Similarly, Robinson's 'Patent' Barley Water urged nurses to use the product 'as a dilutant of milk for infant feeding'.[31] The private nurse was encouraged not only to purchase these products on behalf of the patient, but also to advise him or her as to which product or brand was the most suitable.[32]

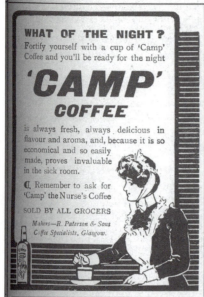
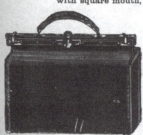
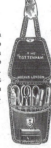
Figure 10.1　Camp, '. . . invaluable in the sick room'. *Nursing Times*, 5 January 1907, p. 7.

'WORKING FOR THE WELFARE OF MOTHERS AND INFANTS': ADVERTISING TO *c.* 1929

From the turn of the twentieth century, emphasis on the need for appropriate methods of infant feeding became a recurring theme in advertisements in nursing periodicals. The political debates about the health of conscripts which had emerged in the aftermath of the Boer War in 1901 had led to a nationwide concern for the health of babies and mothers. The need for British babies to be – literally – fighting fit, was a central tenet of British social welfare in the early part of the century.[33] Nurses (private nurses, public health nurses, district nurses and midwives) were pinpointed as having an important role to play in the nurturing of appropriate infant feeding methods and general infant welfare. [34] Manufacturers were not slow to develop and advertise products that would improve the health of the babies and children of Britain, and they aimed directly at nurses as the intermediaries between manufacturers and mothers. One of the earliest was Aylesbury Dairy Co., which advertised 'Milk and Cream absolutely free from preservatives' and 'humanised milk' in the nursing press by 1903.[35] By 1915, as the need for fit babies grew ever stronger, 'Frame Food, The Economical Body Building Food for Babies and Invalids' declared that 'Frame Food Babies Never Have Rickets'.[36] Similarly, in 1917 Kepler Malt Extract claimed to be 'working for the welfare of mothers and infants'. With the use of Kepler Malt Extract, so the advertisement proclaimed, it would be 'Baby Week every week'.[37]

Throughout the First World War and into the 1920s, advertisements for baby foods grew in volume and developed new techniques of manipulation. In 1914, Virol infant food was one of the earliest to make use of these new methods (Figure 10.2). Inspired by the political propaganda techniques of war time,[38] Virol abandoned the old line drawings and sketches so characteristic of Victorian and Edwardian periodical advertisements, presenting instead emotive 'before taking Virol' and 'after taking Virol' photographs of infants. In one particular example, the former picture of 'Baby Sutton' showed a fretful infant, thin, 'weak and wasted', writhing upon the ground in a passion of agony and despair. The second picture purported to show the same 'Baby Sutton' after having taken Virol for eight months. The child was now plump, smiling and happy. The copy was a combination of different, but fulsome, endorsements. A homely 'thank-you' letter by 'Mrs B. Sutton [of] Brixton' was followed by a paragraph combining a pseudo-scientific discussion about 'elaborate . . . investigations' and 'experiments' conducted with Virol and an insistence on the need for the product for 'children who do not thrive'. The manipulation of emotions – fear, that a child would be in pain, and would waste away or otherwise 'fall prey to the germs that will surely attack', and guilt that failing to use the product meant irresponsible nursing and motherhood – was a technique new to advertising. Such advertisements drew unashamedly upon the prevailing emotional and political climate that the need to preserve infant life was essential to the future of the nation.[39]

From the close of the First World War, advertisements in nursing periodicals changed significantly in content and quality: images became more sophisticated

"was weak and wasted"

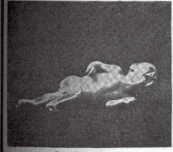
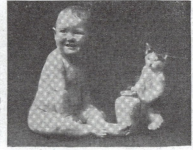

BABY SUTTON   BABY SUTTON

BEFORE TAKING VIROL   AFTER TAKING VIROL

Mrs. B. SUTTON, 4, Akerman Rd., Brixton, writes :—

"When my little daughter was about two months old she did not thrive. Being unable to feed her myself, I tried various infant foods, but none benefited her, and she became so weak and ailing that the doctor was unable to vaccinate her, and I began to fear that I should never be able to bring her up.

"At last I tried Virol. From the first my girl seemed to improve, until now at ten months old she is as fine and bonny a baby as anyone could wish to see."

An elaborate series of investigations recently conducted at a well-known sanatorium has definitely proved that the addition of Virol to the diet exercises a remarkable influence on the phagocytic action of the leucocytes. The experiments showed there was a distinct and progressive increase in the functional activity of the white cells in proportion to the number of weeks the patient had been fed on Virol.

It is, therefore, not surprising that thousands of letters have been written by mothers to say that baby's life was saved by Virol; and the reason is that Virol is compounded of just those foods, largely red bone-marrow itself, which provide the blood-making bones and glands of the body with what they need to help them to maintain the army of white fighting cells.

Virol makes firm flesh, strong bones, and rosy cheeks. Give Virol to children who do not thrive, for they are in a dangerous condition, ready to fall a prey to the germs that will surely attack them.

VIROL

Used in more than 1,000 Hospitals & Sanatoria

VIROL, LTD., 152/166, Old Street, London, E.C.   In jars, at 1/-, 1/8, 2/11.

It is well to mention "The Nursing Times" when answering its Advertisements.

Figure 10.2 Virol, '. . . was weak and wasted'. *Nursing Times*, 1 August 1914, p. 987.

and persuasive techniques developed. From the late 1920s the nurse as consumer increasingly entered the advertisement herself, offering advice or using a product or service and extolling its virtues to her patient or fellow-nurse consumer. The voice in the advertisement became the voice of the nurse, as expert consumer, rather than the voice of the manufacturer simply listing the benefits of that particular product. Social and medical concerns of the day were reflected in the texts and images that were presented in these advertisements, and the role that the nurse, as a professional and as a woman, might have in overcoming such problems was highlighted.

From 1918 products for mothers and babies continued to dominate the advertising pages of the nursing press. Virol had, by the 1920s, repositioned itself as a food for invalids and as an essential preparation for breastfeeding mothers. In the aftermath of war much of the emancipation that women had obtained was rapidly replaced with an emphasis on the need for them to return to the home and to the proper management of their domestic duties.[40] This included a promotion of breastfeeding, as opposed to bottle-feeding, as being 'best' for babies (and therefore best for the nation). In 1914 Virol had been promoted as the ideal milk substitute for babies who were not breast fed. By 1920, however, it was aimed instead at mothers themselves to consume, in order to breastfeed better. 'Virol' ran a series of advertisements throughout the early 1920s in the *Queens Nurses Magazine* – a new journal aimed at district nurses. These advertisements showed photographs of one baby (Baby Peffer), two babies (The Stilwell Twins), and three babies (The Brock Triplets . . . Frank, Cyril and Roy), all of whose mothers had been able to nurse lavishly due to consumption of Virol.[41] In concert with this, and echoing one of the continuing public health concerns of the late 1920s and 1930s, advertisements also acknowledged that '[m]aternal mortality is far higher than it ought to be'. In 1929, for example, an advertisement for Marshall's Lysol Disinfectant drew attention to the role of 'every doctor and nurse . . . in reducing this grave social problem.[42]

RECESSION, ADVERTISING AND THE NURSE ON DUTY

With the post-war recession the role of advertisements as a point of intersection between the aspirations of the nursing profession, the political currents of the time and the demands of the economy became more acute. The addition of photographs and detailed images, and the development of a rhetorical style of copy, allowed a persuasive ideological message to emerge. Although advertising had always circumscribed the most basic concerns and duties of the nurse – promoting starched dresses and caps, accessories, disinfectants, invalid foods and purgatives – it became far more ideologically loaded and prescriptive as the twentieth century proceeded. In many advertisements throughout the period, for instance, the similarities between the duties of the mother and the duties of the nurse were highlighted. Many products, such as King's Patented Cooked Oatmeal, were advertised as 'A boon to mothers and nurses' and 'ideal for Ladies, Invalids and Growing Children' – a telling categorization.[43] The nurse's duties, either in the hospital or in the sick room, were implied to be similar to the duties of the mother in the home, and her relation with the doctor was seen to be similar to the relationship between a mother and a father. She might clean and care, assist in the feeding of children and offer advice on matters of hygiene, but she was always only a helpmate to the doctor.

Throughout the 1920s more and more products were advertising to the nurse in her role as intermediary between bad health and good. Although pharmaceutical products were not advertised to nurses in this period, convalescent foods, beef teas and other restoratives continued to be promoted. By the late 1920s, with the recent discovery of vitamins revolutionizing the way in which human nutrition was understood, the 'preventive aspects of medicine' and the nurse's invaluable role in this found their way into the advertisement pages of the nursing press.[44] In 1923 the persistent makers of Virol drew attention to the important 'vitamine' [sic] content of their product,[45] and preparations designed specifically as 'vitamin food' appeared on the market. Radio-Malt took out a full-page advertisement in 1929 (Figure 10.3). The role of the nurse in administering this 'unique product' was persuasively emphasized. In a rhetorical style familiar in modern advertising, Radio-Malt laid the responsibility for the knowledge and expertise necessary to fully appreciate the product's benefits at the feet of the nurse. The nurse was now able to use a 'scientific product', one in line with the 'trend in modern medicine'. Indeed, as the makers of Radio Malt rather boldly suggested, the preventative work of the nurse was perhaps even more important than the curative work of the doctor.[46]

The image of the nurse as trusted advice-giver was commonplace in advertising from the early 1930s. It was used to promote products from antiseptics and disinfectants to corsets, beef tea and sanitary products.[47] It was baby foods and preparations for the nursing mother, however, which were most often advertised in this way. The nurse, as the fount of advice on matters of health and hygiene, was pinpointed as the main source of communication between the manufacturer and the consumption of numerous 'health giving foods' by (especially) female patients. 'Humanised Trufood, for instance, ran the trite 'Diary of Nurse Bennett' every month throughout 1933 (Figure 10.4). The nun-like Nurse Bennett, who appeared to be dressed in a habit, constantly met babies of great beauty and bigness whom she had introduced to Humanised Trufood when they were new born and 'scarcely alive'.[48] As the advertisements for Trufood indicate, the nurse might recommend but the 'patient' would continue to use the product once the influence of the nurse had been withdrawn. In this way, manufacturers and advertisers made extensive use of advertisements in nurses' journals to get their products to a wider buying public.

Advertisers perceived wives and mothers to be the main holders of the domestic purse strings, and the idea of women as consumers fitted in neatly with the moral and economic climate of the time.[49] Indeed, by the 1930s the world economy had sunk into recession. In response, advertisements sought to encourage the consumer to spend: spending money was patriotic, as it was the only sure way of lifting the economy out of recession.[50] As a result, advertisements

RADIO - MALT

and

'the importance of the preventive aspects of medicine'

THE trend of modern medicine is towards prevention rather than treatment; it is suggested, in effect, that the treatment of disease is of secondary importance in comparison with the prevention of it, and the nurse finds that she is continually being called upon to advise her patients upon the methods of maintaining health.

Acting in the capacity of adviser she will lay stress upon the importance of diet and habits, and will be gratified that there is available a scientific product of the nature of Radio-Malt, inasmuch as it possesses in a remarkable degree the power to raise the resistance of the human body against septic and infective organisms, and is therefore of unique value in combating their attack.

A small daily dose of about a teaspoonful taken during the Autumn and the early Winter will have the effect of building up a reserve of power to withstand the onslaught of infection when colds, influenza and other epidemics of the winter months are rife.

In periods of stress such as in pregnancy, during the physiological changes of puberty and the menopause, and in fact at all times when there is abnormal strain upon the system there is need of just such sustenance as is available through the administration of this unique product.

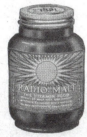

Tasting Sample on request

THE BRITISH DRUG HOUSES LTD.   LONDON N.1

Vit. Pr/Mis. 24

Figure 10.3   Radio-Malt, *Nursing Times*, 28 December 1929, p. 1520.

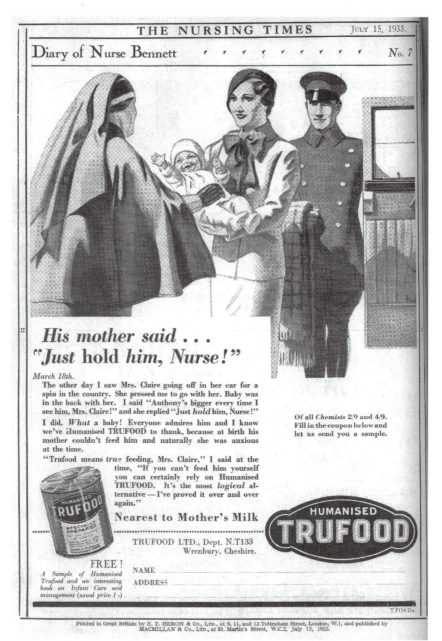

Figure 10.4 Humanised Trufood, diary of Nurse Bennett, *Nursing Times*, 15 July 1933, Cover.

became much more visually sophisticated, with photographs and realistic pictures accompanied by persuasive text becoming increasingly popular. The image of the nurse – always slim, attractive and stylish – began to make more of an appearance, often in a 'realistic' setting. By the beginning of the 1930s a number of long-running advertisements for particular branded products had developed 'scenarios' to situate the product in nurses' lives. These advertisements indicated, through persuasive use of words and images, how the life and work of the nurse might be made easier by the consumption of that particular product. Ovaltine, the 'Tonic Food Beverage' that promised to 'Build up Brain, Nerve and Body', began one such campaign in 1929 (Figure 10.5).[51] Throughout the 1930s Ovaltine showed numerous images of attractive and active nurses in various settings to advertise their product. The Ovaltine nurse – always slender and beautiful – was shown with a nursing mother, going off to work at night and nursing the private patient.[52] She was also depicted studying the list of ingredients on the tin, drinking 'Ovaltine' on a busy ward, dressed in a nun-like head-dress and flourishing a tin of Ovaltine, sharing a cup of 'Ovaltine' with a colleague and with a grateful and beatifically smiling elderly patient.[53]

In addition to advertisements, from the 1930s manufacturers found new ways of promoting their products and brands to the nurse. Sponsorship and public relations made an appearance. In 1937, for example, 'generous gifts for bursaries and scholarships' were made available to the public health nurse 'from Boots Ltd',[54] and in 1938 'seven grants of £5 each were given to members of the [public health nurses] section to enable them to attend the Special Course in Public Health ... at the [Royal] College [of Nursing]'. These grants were made available by manufacturers such as 'Aspro Ltd, Cow and Gate Ltd, Egerton Burnetts Ltd ... [and] Nestles Milk Products Ltd,' all of whom had advertised their products in the nursing press since the 1910s and 1920s. In addition, 'social activities' were organized by these manufacturers, which included such edifying excursions as 'visits to ... Nestle Milk Products condensery in Chippenham.'[55]

HARD SELL: GUILT, FEAR AND THE NURSE OFF DUTY

During the 1930s, patterns of consumption in Britain changed rapidly and radically. Patterns of consumption among nurses, as women of independent means, were no exception. In the earlier part of the century nurses had been notoriously poorly paid – good character and the desire for employment being perceived to be sufficient attributes to encourage recruitment, rather than the incentive of pay. The enormous expansion of hospital facilities that accompanied the First World War, however, had necessitated an increased number of nursing recruits.[56] Furthermore, with the great loss of male lives during the First World War, many women had entered nursing as a career for life. Finally, with standards in women's general education improving, working-class and lower-middle-class women were able to make up an increasingly large proportion of nursing recruits. As a result, the profession became more attractive to a class of young women who might previously have been considered inappropriate for the job.[57] With a disposable

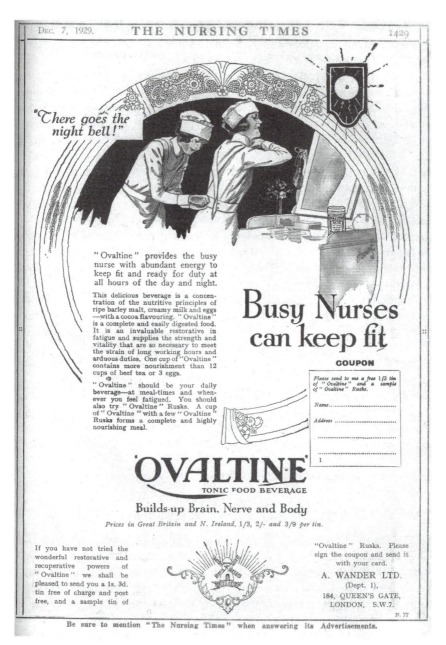

Figure 10.5 Ovaltine, 'busy nurses can keep fit', *Nursing Times*, 7 December 1929, p. 1429.

income that remained consistent despite the vagaries of the post-war economy, by the 1930s nurses were in command of a reasonable salary. As Monica Baly has suggested, 'the staff nurse, with her £50 to £60 a year after all her living needs had been met was not as badly off as has sometimes been depicted'.[58] The private nurse, however, was in a position to earn far greater sums than her institution-bound counterparts. Although 'many hundreds . . . are struggling to make £50 a year,' a great proportion of private nurses were able to earn 'a minimum of £85' per annum, whereas 'the income of the private nurse who has other qualifications besides those of her general training may be from £150 to £200 a year, exclusive of all her expenses'.[59] With such an income, the private nurse was indeed a potentially lucrative consumer. In addition, the emancipation the war had afforded women meant that they were now recognized as reasonable targets for the ever more persuasive techniques of manufacturers and advertisers.

From the mid-1930s the nursing press was advertising hundreds of consumable items that a nurse might possibly need – both as a professional person and as a (lower-middle or working-class) woman. A new journal – *Nursing Illustrated* – sprang up in 1938. It was the most magazine-like of the periodicals tailored specifically for nurses and, in addition to stories, beauty tips and knitting patterns, contained a vast outpouring of advertisements, the like of which had not before appeared in nurses' professional journals. The older, more established journals also joined in the advertising frenzy.

Increasingly, readers were presented with persuasive images and captions pinpointing particular social inadequacies and neuroses to encourage them to buy the products that would ease these social discomforts. Advertisements for personal hygiene products, for example, capitalized on women's fear of smelling badly, a fear especially dreadful for the nurse because of her close proximity to patients. 'In spite of her daily bath' ran the caption for MUM deodorant, 'she's an UNDERARM VICTIM' (capitals in original). 'She's guilty of that greatest social crime – perspiration odour. But before you criticise, are you sure that you never offend in this way?'.[60] Similarly, sanitary products, such as Kotex sanitary pads (the 'modern hygienic necessity'), promised 'perfect safety' and 'longer protection', as well as the ability to 'de-odourise' this basic womanly function.[61] Hosezene sanitary towels offered 'emancipation!!' and the ability to wear 'the thinnest gowns with security'.[62] 'Safety' and the banishment of menstrual odour was also promised by tampon manufacturers, with all 'risk' of 'infection' minimized by this most 'hygienic method of sanitary protection' (although the product was not recommended for 'unmarried girls', who were, presumably, to make do with less hygienic methods until they were fortunate enough to be married).[63] A great proliferation of advertisements for corsets appeared, encouraging one to be 'SURE of healthy slimness' and 'guaranteed to beautify your figure in 10 days'. The growth of credit and higher purchase ensured that the reader could buy the product 'in only 5 monthly instalments of 2/-'.[64] Women appeared in increasingly glamorous and suggestive poses modelling coats, 'autumn and winter fashions' 'frocks' and underwear.

Nurses' private lives and their professional performance also came under the scrutiny of the advertiser's gaze. An advertisement for Norwich Union Pensions depicted a young, made-up nurse, who was 'independent now'. Next to this, a picture of a worried looking elderly lady carrying a handful of drooping flowers asked 'at 55 will you *still* be independent?'[65] Advertisements for beauty products also began to make their appearance. Max Factor offered nurses the chance to look 'Gloriously beautiful' like Loretta Young through a 'personal complexion analysis', and Pears invited the nurse to transform 'dull sluggish skin' to a 'new loveliness … which every woman envies'.[66] Advertisements also informed nurses that they had performed their duties badly and failed exams because they had not 'learned how success is won the night before' by drinking Bourn-vita.[67] Throughout the late 1920s and 1930s, guilt – of not being a good mother; of not being patriotic enough to buy the 'British made' item; fear – of disease and uncleanliness, of infant death, of having body odour or menstrual leakages; of being fat and unshapely; of not being 'lovely'; of failing one's exams or of losing one's independence in old age, were emotions that were increasingly preyed upon by advertisers to compel the nurse to buy more and more products aimed at enhancing her security, her looks or her performance at work.

By the late 1930s, advertisements portrayed the nurse not only as a serious health professional but also as a young, emancipated individual with a vibrant social life, the time and money to shop and pursue outdoor activities, and a 'duty' to look slim and attractive both in and out of work. The range of consumer products on which the nurse was encouraged to spend her income also expanded at an unprecedented rate. Advertisements for motorbikes and pushbikes made their appearance in 1938;[68] whereas advertisements for products specifically associated with holidays, socializing and off-duty time also entered the pages of nursing journals.[69] Craven 'A' cigarettes were advertised picturing a glamorous young woman smiling coquettishly upwards with a half-smoked cigarette smouldering between painted fingers.[70] New advertisements such as these ran along side longstanding advertisements for Garrould's Complete Nurse Outfitters, Brands Beef Essence and California Syrup of Figs.

NURSING, CONSUMPTION AND IDEOLOGY

From this period, advertisements in nurses' journals also mirrored more subtle changes in society and in the nurse's professional role. The language and images of advertisements suggest that an ideological shift at the level of the consumer occurred. Consumption itself, in addition to caring for the sick, was now seen as a productive activity for nurses. In addition, throughout the 1930s, women were encouraged to return to the home to fulfil their natural social duties. For the nurse, the moral tenor of the 1930s advocated strength of character in the performance of like duties in the sick room, and in the regulation of environmental and bodily hygiene. Nurses were encouraged, through advertising, to accommodate new 'scientific insights' in hygiene and childcare, new food brands and new innovations in cleanliness in her professional life, as well as in her personal life and in the lives of her patients. Thus, as the nurse made the sick room well ordered and hygienic through the purchase and use of certain products, so the well-ordered and smooth functioning of the body mirrored these regimes. Advertisements for laxatives were perhaps the most widespread of all advertisements that appeared in nurses' periodicals throughout the inter-war period. 'Torpid bowels' it was noted, resulted in all manner of ailments, especially in women, including 'congestion of the uterus . . . functional disorders . . . and even inflammatory conditions'.[71] From the early 1930s almost every journal contained promotional material advocating at least one brand of laxative. The benefits of a regular, and orderly, evacuation were manifold and advertisements frequently contained lavish descriptions of the 'lubricating', 'easing' and 'final expulsion' of the offending matter.[72] The nurse was represented as an authority figure in the choice and administration of the appropriate brand and dose. Magnolax, Purgoids, Innerclean, Agarol, Medilax, Eno's Fruit Salts, Andrew's Liver Salts, Petrol-Agar, Dinneford's, Lixen, Californian Syrup of Figs, Shredded Wheat, Kellogg's All Bran and Weetabix were just some of the brands on offer to combat the 'menace of the overloaded bowel'.[73]

Perhaps the most interesting aspect of advertising generally during the Second World War is the great shift that occurred in the image of women. From the outbreak of war in 1939, women were increasingly portrayed fixing machinery, driving buses and generally engaged in other, formerly manly, pursuits.[74] Although nurses had always been 'working women', from 1939 they were only one group of many women who now did paid, often manual, work for a living. The idea of the nurse as a professional individual with manifold serious medical roles to perform, however, was overshadowed by the domestic images presented in advertisements. Rather than nurses taking on men's jobs, their profession was seen as an extension of their traditional womanly role as carer and sickbed attendant. As a result, advertisements continued to portray the nurse feeding infants (or at least advising mothers on the subject), and cleaning wards and bedrooms – or, at least, she was urged to acquire the products that would allow her to do so.[75] Clearly, the links between women's distinctly 'feminine' role in the home, and her 'feminine' role as a nurse or 'angel' were maintained, and reinforced, through the messages of war time advertising.

In addition, the outbreak of war and the acknowledgement of the nurse's working role in society did not prevent the emergence of an even greater number of advertisements for beauty products – corsets, make-up and fashionable dresses – from appearing in the nursing press. Such advertisements reminded the nurse that it was now her duty, as the raiser of morale at the bedside and as the source of 'charming company' to servicemen, to look better than ever. 'Nowadays, beauty is a duty, since it cheers and inspires yourself and others', declared an advertisement for Insta Pak beauty cream.[76] Pictures of servicemen began to make their appearance as the objects of nurses' attention (both as patients and as the objects of nurses' off-duty charms).[77] Nurses were described as 'very busy but very lovely' or 'rushed, but radiant'. As P and B knitting wools observed, 'it isn't going to help anybody if you let go of your appearance'.[78] Indeed, advertisements stressed that the nurse was required, by the very nature of her profession, 'to bring courage and support to the lives of those about you' and her appearance was emphasized as being essential to this morale-boosting role.[79] The hands, skin, hair and body of the nurse were all now constantly under the critical gaze of advertising.[80] No longer was efficiency on the job and the physical health of patients seen to be the direct primary aim of nursing, but the social pressures of attractiveness and of not 'letting go of one's appearance' emerged as vital aspects of the caring role. Advertising in this period, therefore, played a complex part in reinforcing women's concerns about their appearance. For the nurse, her appearance was medicalized, with attention to face and figure portrayed as a form of psychological therapy vital for the recovery of her patients. In a language reminiscent of that used to describe the Bovril and Oxo brands of beef tea in the 1890s, advertisements proceeded to stress that a 'lovely' nurse was a 'tonic' and 'restorative' to 'those around her'.[81]

CONCLUSION

This brief study has indicated ways in which advertising in nursing periodicals developed to become a sophisticated vehicle for the promotion of products in response to the political and social impulses of the time. National concern for the health of mothers and babies, for example, was reflected in the type of products advertised, and also in the language used in those advertisements. From the 1920s, as women were encouraged to return to the home to fulfil their domestic and procreative duties after the war, this too was echoed in the language and images of advertising. The nurse – especially the private, district or public health nurse – was a key figure in encouraging women to stay at home and to breast-feed, and this role was reflected in the products advertised in the nursing press in this period. Furthermore, as women gained more autonomy and greater freedom in society, so advertisements in nurses' professional journals mirrored these changes. Products for the nurse to use on her holidays or in her leisure time increased, and the image of the nurse herself became more modern. Nurses were shown riding bicycles, wearing swimming costumes and using cosmetics. However, despite the 'emancipation' (as one advertisement described it)[82] that consumerism afforded nurses, one theme that comes across strongly in the study is the extent to which advertising imprisoned the nurse within an ideology of femininity, both in her professional duties and, by the early 1940s, also in her physical appearance.

Although a far greater level of analysis remains to be done, the above discussion has drawn attention to a much-overlooked aspect of nursing and medical history – the emergence of the nurse as consumer. It has also provided an insight into the way in which advertisements portrayed the nurse – as carer at the bedside, as advisor of mothers, unblocker of bowels, and the owner of the slim, cool and 'lovely' hand laid on the patient's brow.

The impact of advertising images on society, as well as on particular professional groups, is complex and profound. As Kalisch and Kalisch have observed, 'every mirror has some effect on the behaviour of those who look into it'.[83] Whether these images showed the nurse as she was, as she aspired to be or as medicine and society thought she ought to be, is also a subject requiring further discussion.

NOTES

1   E. Goffman, *Gender Advertisements*, London: Macmillan, 1979; R. Goldman, *Reading Ads Socially*, London: Routledge, 1992; J. Williamson, *Decoding Advertisements: Ideologies and Meaning in Advertising*, London: Boyars, 1978; M. A. Masse and K. Rossenblum, 'Male and female, they created them: the depiction of gender in the advertising of traditional women's and men's magazines,' *Women's Studies International Forum*, 1998, Vol. 11, pp. 124–44.

2   R. Goldman, 'Marketing fragrances: advertising and the production of commodity signs', *Theory, Culture and Society*, 1987, Vol. 4, pp. 691–725; G. Myers, *Words in Ads*, London: Arnold, 1994; R. Barthes, *Mythologies*, London: Jonathan Cape Ltd, 1972; R. Goldman and S. Papson, 'Advertising in the age of hypersignification,' *Theory, Culture and Society*, 1994, Vol. 11, pp. 23–53.

3   R. Ohmann, *Selling Culture: Magazines, Markets and Class at the Turn of the Century*, London: Verso, 1998; F. Mort, *Cultures of Consumption: Masculinities and Social Space in Late Twentieth-century Britain*, London: Routledge, 1996; J. Berger, *Ways of Seeing*, London: Penguin, 1972.

4   V. Packard, *The Hidden Persuaders*, London: Penguin, 1981; S. Otnes and L. Scott, 'Something old, something new: exploring the interaction between ritual and advertising', *Journal of Advertising*, 1996, Vol. 25, pp. 25–31; B. Stern, 'Gender and multicultural issues in advertising: stages in the research highway', *Journal of Advertising*, 1999, Vol. 28, pp. 1–9.

5   Ohmann, *Selling Culture*, p. 11.

6   Berger, *Ways of Seeing*, pp. 129–34.

7   Williamson, *Decoding Advertisements*, p. 13.

8   P. Kalisch and B. Kalisch, *The Changing Image of the Nurse*, California: Addison-Wesley, 1987, p. 2.

9   Goffman, *Gender Advertisements*; I. Mayne, 'The inescapable images: gender and advertising', *Equal Opportunities International*, 2000, Vol. 19, pp. 56–61.

10 See, for example, C. M. Chapman, 'Image of the nurse', *International Nursing Review*, 1977, Vol. 24, pp. 166–70; J. Bridges, 'Literature review of images of the nurse and nursing in the media', *Journal of Advanced Nursing*, 1990, Vol. 15, pp. 850–4; A. H. Jones, *Images of Nurses: Perspectives from History, Art and Popular Culture*, Philadelphia: University of Pennsylvania Press, 1988; Kalisch and Kalisch, *Changing Image*.

11 J. Hallam, *Nursing the Image: Media, Culture and Professional Identity*, London: Routledge, 2000, pp. 84–129.

12 L.A. Loeb, *Consuming Angels: Advertising and Victorian Women*, Oxford: Oxford University Press, 1994; C. Davies, *Gender and the Professional Predicament in Nursing*, Buckingham: Open University Press, 1995; D. Wicks, *Doctors and Nurses at Work: Rethinking Professional Boundaries*, London: Open University Press, 1998.

13 D.A. Leslie, 'Femininity, post-Fordism and the "new traditionalism" ', in L. McDowell and J. P. Sharp (eds), *Space, Gender, Knowledge: Feminist Readings*, London: Routledge, 1997, pp. 300–17.

14 Kalisch, *Changing image*, p. x; K. Myers, *Understains: the Sense and Seduction of Advertising*, London: Open University Press, 1998, pp. 4–6.

15 R. Dingwall, A. M. Rafferty and C. Webster, *An Introduction to the Social History of Nursing*, London: Routledge, 1988, pp. 68–72.

16 Annual reports of the Royal College of Nursing, 1931–1938.

17 Marianne Wenden, *Private Nursing*, London: Faber and Faber, 1936, p. ix.

18 Margaret Breay, 'How can private nurses keep in touch with modern methods?' *The Nursing Record and Hospital World*, 1897, Vol. 18, p. 232.

19 Wenden, *Private Nursing*, pp. 43 and 49. Wenden goes on to list a whole range of products, most of which are brand names, which the private nurse may find of use. All are advertised in the nursing press.

20 Ibid., pp. 97–9.

21 Breay, 'How can private nurses keep in touch', p. 232

22 Images often had little to do with the product in question. In 1892, for instance, an advertisement in the *Nurses Journal* for 'Aperient Water' showed a full-page line drawing of an exotically dressed young woman sipping from a champagne glass, which presumably contained the laxative in question. At the foot of the picture the reader was informed that 'Nurses who would like an exquisitely coloured and enlarged copy of the above photographic facsimile for framing can have one free of charge by post' by writing to the manufacturers. See *Nurses Journal*, 1892, Vol. 2, p. 29.

23 Wenden, *Private Nursing*, pp. 49–50

24 *Nursing Notes*, 1895, Vol. 8, p. 86; *Nursing Record*, 1892, Vol. 8, pp. 34, 357.

25 *Nursing Times*, 1909, Vol. 5, p. 386. See also *Nursing Notes*, 1892, Vol. 5, p. 119; *Nursing Notes*, 1908, Vol. 21, p. 43.

26 Wenden, *Private Nursing*, p. 43

27 *Nurses Journal*, 1892, Vol. 2, p. 29; *Nursing Times*, 1909, Vol. 5, p. 59.

28 *Nursing Times*, 1907, Vol. 3, p. 17.

29 Frontispiece, *Nursing Notes*, 1896, Vol. 9, np. Similarly, the nurse reader was exhorted to 'fortify yourself against the influenza by a liberal use of BOVRIL', *Nursing Record*, 1892, Vol. 8, p. 22, and in 1907 to 'reinforce the system' against the same infection with 'Oxo'. *Nursing Times,* 1907, Vol. 3, p. 17.

30 *Nursing Notes*, 1893, Vol. 6, p. 98.

31 *Nursing Times*, 1909, Vol. 5, p. 593.

32 Wenden, *Private Nursing*, pp. 48–9 and 98–100.

33 See, for example, A. Davin, 'Imperialism and motherhood', *History Workshop,* 1987, Vol. 5, pp. 9–65; C. Dyhouse, 'Working-class mothers and infant mortality in England, 1895–1914,' *Journal of Social History,* 1987, Vol. 12, pp. 248–67; D. Dwork, *War is Good for Babies and Other Young Children: a History of the Infant and Child Welfare Movement in England, 1898–1918*, London/New York: Tavistock, 1987; Jane Lewis, 'The working-class wife and mother and state intervention, 1870–1918,' in Jane Lewis (ed.), *Labour and Love: Women's Experience of Home and Family, 1850–1940*, Oxford: Basil Blackwell, 1986, pp. 99–120.

34 Ibid., pp. 99–104.

35 *Nursing Notes*, 1903, Vol. 16, p. 179.

36 *Nursing Times*, 1915, Vol. 11, p. 138.

37 *Nursing Notes*, 1917, Vol. 30, p. 121.

38 Myers, *Understains,* p. 22.

39 *Nursing Times*, 1914, Vol. 10, p. 987.

40 Anna Davin, Carol Dyhouse and Jane Lewis have all persuasively argued that the 'cult of motherhood' that emerged in the early twentieth century blamed incompetent mothers for the high rate of infant mortality. It was aimed at the social control and repression of women through an emphasis on a notion of their traditional duties, which had its origins in the nineteenth century. All three scholars point to the medical profession as being one of the key players in the struggle to keep women in the home looking after their children. See n. 33 above for references. Dwork attempts to revise the conclusions of these scholars by suggesting that government officials must, surely, have been more concerned with saving babies than with controlling women, and that the importance of poverty was recognized by such officials. See Dwork, *War is Good for Babies*, pp. 228–9.

41 *Queens Nurses Magazine*, 1920–1924. Similarly, 'Glaxo: The Super-Milk' was advertised as the ideal product for mothers to imbibe in order to 'improve their milk from the first day they take it'. *Nursing Times*, 1921, Vol. 17, p. 34.

42 *Nursing Times*, 1929, Vol. 25, p. 173.

43 *Nursing Times*, 1921, Vol. 17, p. 1234.

44 *Nursing Times*, 1929, Vol. 25, p. 1520.

45 *Queens Nurses Magazine*, 1920–1924.
46 *Nursing Times*, 1929, Vol. 25, p. 1520.
47 *Nursing Illustrated*, 1939, Vol. 2, p. 298; *Nursing Illustrated*, 21 October 1938, Vol. 1, no. 7, p. 24; *Nursing Illustrated*, 1939, Vol. 2, p. 370; *Nursing Illustrated*, 1939, Vol. 2, p. 882.
48 January to December *Nursing Times*, 1933, Vol. 29.
49 J. Benson, *The rise of Consumer Society in Britain, 1880–1980*, London: Longman, 1994, p. 180.
50 Myers, 1998, *Understains: the Sense and Seduction*, pp. 24–6.
51 In this advertisement, beneath the exclamation '[t]here goes the night bell!' a young, slim nurse struggled anxiously to help an equally attractive colleague fasten herself into her uniform. To the left, the 'night bell' rings furiously, and the whole scene seems fraught and hurried. A tin of Ovaltine, the only thing in the picture that is not moving, sits calmly on the dressing table. *Nursing Times*, 1929, Vol. 25, p. 1429.
52 *Nursing Notes*, 1930, Vol. 42, p. xlii; *Nursing Notes*, 1 November 1930, Vol. 42, p. lxxviii; *Nursing Notes*, 1 April 1932, Vol. 45, p. cxxxvii.
53 *Nursing Notes*, 1 May 1932, Vol. 45, p. clx; *Nursing Notes*, 1932, Vol. 45, p. clxix; *Nursing Illustrated*, 1938, Vol. 1, no. 1, p. 10; *Nursing Illustrated*, 7 October 1938 Vol. 1, no. 1, p. vi.
54 Royal College of Nursing Annual Report 1937, p. 14.
55 Royal College of Nursing Annual Report 1938, pp. 13–14.
56 M. E. Baly, *Nursing and Social Change*, 3rd edn, London: Routledge, 1995, pp. 156–65.
57 Ibid.
58 Ibid., p. 159.
59 Wenden, *Private Nursing*, pp. 28–29.
60 *Nursing Illustrated*, 1938, Vol. 1, no. 2, p. 6.
61 *Nursing Notes*, 1931, Vol. 44, p. iv.
62 *Nursing Notes*, 1932, Vol. 45, p. 360.
63 *Nursing Illustrated*, 1938, Vol. 1, no. 3, p. 52.
64 *Nursing Illustrated*, 1938, Vol. 1, no. 12, p. v.
65 *Nursing Illustrated*, 1938, Vol. 1, no. 8, p. 8. It is interesting to note that private nurses were retired at 55 (see J. Burdett, *Hospitals and Charities*, London: Faber, 1928, pp. 697–704). The importance of health insurance and pensions for private nurses was stressed in the minutes of the Private Nurses' Committee of the Royal College of Nursing throughout the 1930s, to the extent that a special feature on the subject was commissioned by the College in 1935 to appear in *Nursing Times*. See *Nursing Times*, 1935, Vol. 31, pp. 245–6 (Royal College of Nursing Private Nurses Committee Minutes, 5 November 1934, no pagination). Note also that *Nursing Times* was the official organ of the Royal College of Nursing. In the 1930s, the income from advertisements enabled the College to 'share in the journal's profits.' (Annual Report of the Royal College of Nursing, 1934, p. 3).
66 *Nursing Illustrated*, 1938, Vol. 1, no. 12, p. xi.
67 *Nursing Illustrated*, 1938, Vol. 1, no. 1, p. 54.
68 *Nursing Illustrated*, 1939, Vol. 2, p. 588.
69 In June and July of 1939 *Nursing Illustrated* contained a series of advertisements for 'nurses seeking a really super holiday'. Holiday camps and motoring holidays were advertised to accompany a two-part article about holiday destinations. See *Nursing Times*, 1938, Vol. 34, p. 347.
70 *Nursing Illustrated*, 1939, Vol. 2, p. 882.
71 *Nursing Illustrated*, 1938, Vol. 1, no. 9, p. 65.
72 Ibid.
73 *Nursing Notes*, 1930, Vol. 42, p. xii. Almost all of these products offered a 'liberal trial quantity free to nurses on request'. Furthermore, the nurse was frequently expected

'to recommend it to patients', thereby ensuring ever greater sales. See, for example, *Nursing Illustrated*, 1938, Vol. 1, no. 1, p. xiv. The private nurse was urged to offer 'advice with regard to aperients' particularly to her female patients, 'in case the patient has not mentioned the existence of constipation when consulting her doctor.' See Wenden, *Private nursing*, p. 97.

74   *Midwives Chronicle and Nursing Notes*, 1942, Vol. 55, p. xxiv; *Midwives Chronicle and Nursing Notes*, 1943, Vol. 56, p. xxiii.
75   *Midwives Chronicle and Nursing Notes*, 1944, Vol. 57, p. 109; *Midwives Chronicle and Nursing Notes*, 1945, Vol. 58, p. 27.
76   *Nursing Illustrated*, 1939, Vol. 2, p. 886.
77   *Nursing Illustrated*, 1939, Vol. 2. p. 26; *Nursing Illustrated*, 1940, Vol. 4, p. 340.
78   *Nursing Illustrated*, 10 May 1940, Vol. 4, p. 56.
79   Ibid.
80   *Nursing Illustrated*, 1939, Vol. 3, p. 364; *Nursing Illustrated*, 1940, Vol. 3, p. 538; *Nursing Illustrated*, 1940, Vol. 3, p. 36.
81   Despite this emphasis on personal beauty, however, and the cry 'Nurses . . . look your best,' the cosmetically enhanced nurse was urged to draw upon 'dignity and restraint because of their noble profession' when applying make up, especially in case of 'upsetting superiors'. *Nursing Illustrated*, 1939, Vol. 2, p. 885.
82   *Nursing Notes*, November 1932, Vol. 45, p. 360.
83   Kalisch and Kalisch, *Changing Image*, p. 4.

11 Exploring the maternity archive of the St Helens Hospital, Wellington, New Zealand, 1907–22

An historian and midwife collaborate

Pamela J. Wood and Maralyn Foureur

In response to a growing concern about New Zealand's maternal and infant mortality rates at the beginning of the twentieth century, the 1904 Midwives Act established formal midwifery training and registration, and enabled the setting up of St Helens Hospitals throughout New Zealand. From the establishment of the first four in 1905, these hospitals provided both maternity care for married women whose husbands earned less than £3 a week and a training place for midwives. By 1920, seven hospitals had been set up and, although the criteria for admission changed over time, St Helens Hospitals provided a safe maternity service for New Zealand women for the next seven decades. The hospitals are historically interesting for three main reasons: (i) they provide a very early example of state-subsidized maternity hospitals in the international twentieth-century context; (ii) the majority of births were attended only by midwives and maternity nurses; and (iii) the hospitals led New Zealand on all indices of safe maternity care.[1] St Helens Hospitals were therefore a site of significant development in midwifery practice and maternity services in New Zealand.

The Wellington St Helens Hospital was the first one established, in May 1905. Following the discovery of the records of this hospital in 2000, a detailed analysis is now possible of its birth-related records. The archive comprises fifty-seven volumes, chiefly casebooks, admission books and maternity registers, from 1907 until the hospital's closure in 1980. The archive has two almost continuous runs: the first from 1907 until 1922, the second from 1929 until 1980. These allow a fairly comprehensive analysis of changes in the demographic profile and delivery histories of women who gave birth at St Helens over seven decades. This chapter offers preliminary findings from an analysis of the first run. Although records are incomplete for the years 1907, 1910, 1911 and 1922, the remaining 3,166 records provide an extensive sample and rich source of information. Other primary sources, such as official government reports, offer material to enable the St Helens data to be contextualized.

In addition, this study enables two researchers with differing clinical and research backgrounds to collaborate in a new way. Our differing interests in nursing history, on the one hand, and epidemiology and clinical midwifery, on the other, allow us to address both historical and current clinical issues through information yielded by the archive.

This chapter explores the nature of our collaboration and how different perspectives assist with the analysis of complex issues. Examples of our preliminary findings are presented to illustrate the kinds of enquiry that are possible using the material contained in these records. The first example provides baseline demographic information about the population of women who gave birth at St Helens Hospital Wellington, 1907–22, and considers in particular the issue of maternal mortality. The other two examples describe lines of enquiry we are exploring concerned with the way in which women's bodies were inscribed by the birth process: perineal tears, sutures and the question of episiotomy, and the descriptive gaze applied to the women's breasts. To understand the context of the St Helens Hospital, a brief description is first provided of the development of this new maternity service.

ST HELENS HOSPITALS

Although no detailed history of the St Helens Hospitals has been written, historians have referred to them in considering different aspects of maternity in New Zealand.[2] St Helens Hospitals were named after the Lancashire birthplace of Richard John Seddon, the New Zealand Premier 1893–1906, who took a keen political interest in maternal welfare. The initiative for them, however, came from a different source. Grace Neill, a Scottish-born English-trained nurse who was the government's Assistant Inspector of Hospitals, urged Seddon to establish hospitals that could provide safe maternity care for women who could not afford private care in a hospital or their home, as well as offering a site for training midwives. In 1901 Neill had drafted legislation for the registration and regulation of nurses. Three years later, she argued the case for a Midwives Act and this scheme of state-controlled maternity hospitals. Her persuasiveness convinced Seddon not only of the case, which fitted well with his concerns for maternal welfare and his own working-class background, but also that Neill should personally oversee the establishment of the first hospital. It was at Neill's suggestion that the hospitals were named after his birthplace, perhaps an inspired idea to ensure his support.[3]

Plans for the state maternity hospitals were finalized in 1905 and the first St Helens Hospital opened in June in a rented house in Rintoul Street, Newtown, a working-class area of Wellington, and close to the public hospital.[4] By 31 March 1906, 111 women had given birth at the hospital.[5] Further St Helens Hospitals opened in 1905 in the other main cities of Auckland, Christchurch and Dunedin, and in later years in the smaller towns of Wanganui, Gisborne and Invercargill. Although using rented houses or altering hastily purchased existing houses enabled the first hospitals to be opened quickly, the accommodation was not ideal and the hospitals gradually shifted to purpose-built premises.[6]

The St Helens Hospitals serve as an early example of the state intervening in the provision of maternity care to assist those who could not afford private care and to improve standards and therefore outcomes. By the late nineteenth century, New Zealand had gained a reputation among international commentators and observers as an effective 'social laboratory', with its legislation for women's franchise, working conditions in factories and workshops, industrial conciliation and arbitration processes, and welfare initiatives. It is therefore not surprising that this initiative for a state maternity service could be implemented relatively quickly.

The St Helens Hospitals also offer an historical model of a maternity service delivered by midwives. A doctor was appointed for each hospital as medical superintendent, with responsibility for general oversight, reporting to government and providing lectures to the training midwives, and it is likely that they influenced service delivery through determining policy and protocol. Doctors like Henry Jellett in the Department of Health, and T. F. Corkhill in private practice, also wrote textbooks for those undertaking midwifery training.[7] In day-to-day terms, however, the doctor was called into the hospital only to attend cases with potential or actual complications.

The Department of Health extended its control over midwifery practice in St Helens Hospitals during the 1920s, introducing reforms to address the significant national maternal mortality problem. An example was the implementation of a strict policy regarding aseptic technique and the extension of antenatal care, under the direction of the Department's doctors, T. L. Paget, Jellett and Elaine Gurr.[8] The hospitals enabled the Department to argue the effectiveness of its policies to resistant doctors in general and private practice. When better outcomes could be demonstrated for St Helens Hospitals, changes in practice could be enlisted elsewhere. This was particularly so in regard to measures designed to reduce puerperal sepsis and forceps deliveries in the 1920s and 1930s.[9]

The St Helens Hospitals therefore serve as a useful example of changing maternity practices within a state-controlled service. This chapter offers some preliminary findings from our analysis of records from one of these hospitals, in relation to the attempt to provide a safe maternity service for working-class women.

Women who gave birth: a demographic profile

From a clinical point of view, maternal age, parity, social class and ethnicity are interrelating and interacting socio-demographic factors that influence maternal health and childbearing. Analysis of the St Helens records in relation to demographic variables therefore has relevance for epidemiologists and midwives concerned with providing a safe service for women today, and for historians interested in how these factors affected a specific group of women in the past.

This analysis is also interesting from an epidemiological view because several factors that might influence birth outcomes are controlled in what can be regarded as a 'natural experiment'. To elaborate: only working-class women were eligible to attend St Helens. All St Helens midwives were trained under a standard system that emphasized asepsis to prevent infection. The midwives did not attend non-maternity patients, so were not exposed to potential colonization by pathogens that they could have passed on to women in their care. No medical student training occurred at St Helens in these years, and no doctors were permitted to admit women there, therefore no additional medical personnel attended women other than the medical superintendent called in for emergencies. It can be described as hospital-based, predominantly midwife-delivered maternity care, provided to one particular social class of women. The database contains all the birth outcomes including cases where the doctor was called. This provides a unique opportunity to examine a number of competing hypotheses about the quality of midwifery practice, location for birth and maternity care outcomes.

The database includes information about 3,166 women who were admitted to the St Helens Hospital, Wellington between 1907 and 1922. Most came to give birth there but others were admitted after giving birth at home. The numbers admitted annually increased gradually over the years to a peak of 330 in 1917. Adjusting for the years with incomplete records, the annual average of 243.41 women at Wellington St Helens represents less than 1 per cent of all births in New Zealand, as the country had on average 27,361 births annually in this time period. As Mein Smith has noted, during this period most women gave birth at home or in small, unlicensed one-bed homes run by a nurse or midwife. In 1920 approximately 65 per cent of births were outside hospitals, with four per cent at the various St Helens Hospitals.[10]

Maternal age

The median age of women admitted to the hospital during this period was twenty-seven years, with a range from twelve to fifty-three years. This is not dissimilar to the median age of twenty-nine years for all New Zealand women giving birth in 1999.[11] The age distribution is also comparable. In 1999, 58 per cent of New Zealand births were to women between the ages of twenty-five and thirty-four years. In the St Helens Wellington group, 50.3 per cent of births were to women in this age group. A further 15.7 per cent of women were aged over thirty-five at St Helens compared with 16.7 per cent in 1999. There were fewer under the age of twenty giving birth at St Helens (3.8 per cent) than in New Zealand in 1999 (7 per cent). A careful analysis of changes in age over the seven decades, however, is needed.

Almost all of the women have been recorded under the title 'Mrs' (99.7 per cent). We do know from the ages of the mothers, however, that some were under the legal age of marriage. This might therefore have been a 'courtesy' title in keeping with the social mores of the time and as such obscures our understanding of the marital status of the women. Unlike today in maternity services, ethnicity was not recorded.

Gravidity and parity

The number of pregnancies each woman had experienced (gravidity) ranged from one to twenty, with the average being 2.75 (SD 2.16) and with 34.1 per cent having their first baby. In New Zealand today, parity refers to the number of times a woman has given birth to an infant, dead or alive, after twenty weeks' gestation or weighing 400 grams or more. Between 1907 and 1922, the definition of parity differed and a 'viable birth' was one occurring after twenty-eight weeks' gestation. Those not considered viable were not included when calculating a woman's parity. In addition, information entered under the heading 'Pregnancies' in the St Helens records probably referred to gravidity rather than parity, although we cannot be sure. For both these reasons, comparisons of current and historical figures are fraught.

There were 519 women (25.3 per cent) who would today be described as 'grand multipara', women having their fourth or subsequent baby. Today this is considered to be associated with an increased risk of complications, including post-partum haemorrhage.[12] Our current understanding of the nature of risk associated with high parity has been largely influenced by the outcomes for such women during the late nineteenth and early twentieth centuries. One of our future tasks will therefore be to explore the outcomes for each group of women (primipara, multipara and grand multipara) to determine the types of risk they faced and their outcomes. Having more specific information could help show whether this understanding of risk is based on credible evidence.

Perinatal deaths

It is not possible to determine an accurate perinatal mortality rate because of the differences over time in the definition of the viability of a fetus. The perinatal mortality rate for New Zealand in 1999 (the latest year for which figures are available) is 10.7 per 1,000 live births. By whatever criteria we could use, it is apparent that the perinatal (infant) mortality at St Helens Wellington – 32.8/1,000 for this period – was much higher than the current figure. However, this rate was much lower than for New Zealand as a whole during the 1907–22 period.[13] This contributed to the confidence in St Helens Hospitals as being some of the safest places to give birth in New Zealand during that time.

MATERNAL DEATHS

Twenty-one women died in this population of 3,166, which equates to a maternal mortality rate of 6.6 per 1,000 live births (or 66.3/10,000). This is extraordinarily high when compared with the rate in New Zealand today of 0.7/10,000 (usually cited as 7/100,000). Maternal mortality figures for New Zealand were not routinely published in the official annual reports of this period but the national rate of 6.48/1,000 in 1920 sparked official alarm and led to a vigorous and contentious campaign to deal with its chief cause, puerperal sepsis, in the ensuing decades.[14]

One hypothesis examined recently by Loudon[15] and by others during the late nineteenth and twentieth centuries[16] is that the type of birth attendant influenced the rate of maternal mortality. In normal births where women were attended predominantly by doctors, the maternal mortality rate was higher than where women were attended by midwives.[17] Loudon cites the New Zealand 1920 maternal mortality rate of 64.8/10,000 births, with the usual attendant at normal births noted as being 'predominantly doctors'.[18] Jellett had proposed in 1929 that the countries with the lowest rates of maternal mortality were those where normal cases were delivered by midwives (Denmark, 1920, 23.5; The Netherlands, 1920, 24.2; Sweden, 1918, 25.8; Norway, 1919, 29.7).[19] In other studies cited by Loudon (for example the Queen's Institute Nurse Midwives, 1905–31), maternal mortality rates for midwives attending women at home were half those of the country as a whole.[20] If this hypothesis were to be supported, one might expect to find lower mortality rates for women giving birth at St Helens, because midwives were the usual attendants at normal birth. However, the evidence for our time period supports neither Loudon's nor Jellett's argument. The maternal mortality rate at St Helens Wellington, 1907–12, was 66.3/10,000, similar to the national rate under predominantly medical care.[21]

The second hypothesis explored by Loudon is that maternal mortality was highest in women from the higher social classes, the rationale being that they were more likely to be attended by doctors. Again the St Helens records do not appear to support this proposal unreservedly. The maternal mortality rate for the working-class women was the same as for New Zealand as a whole. This is offered cautiously as further analysis is needed to make a comparison between rates in private hospitals caring for women from higher social classes. One such hospital, the 'highly respectable' Kelvin Private Maternity Hospital in Auckland, reported five maternal deaths due to puerperal sepsis in 1923, which sparked a crisis of confidence in New Zealand's obstetrical services. The fact that the outbreak 'struck without respect for class or income', implied that women confined by doctors in the 'better' private hospitals had more to fear than working-class wives who gave birth at St Helens Hospitals. A subsequent inquiry defended the doctors but did acknowledge that such outbreaks could only be contained by establishing higher standards of practice for all hospitals.[22]

Most deaths recorded in the St Helens Wellington records indicate women died of conditions unrelated to puerperal sepsis.[23] The women had succumbed to eclampsia or haemorrhage, or as a consequence of a general state of debilitation prior to labour. This finding is of relevance to the third of Loudon's hypotheses to be considered. Many homebirth advocates have argued that history has revealed that the place of birth influenced maternal mortality, with more women dying in hospital than at home. Loudon argues, however, that it is not the place of birth that makes the difference but the type of birth attendant. As doctors were more exposed to non-maternity patients they carried infections, which they then passed on to their maternity clients. Fewer doctors attended women at home, therefore fewer women who gave birth at home died. Again the St Helens records question this assumption. Doctors were rarely present at the births, few women died of puerperal infections but nevertheless the same proportion of women died. In this case it would appear that the health status of the mother might have been a major contributing factor to the women's deaths. A future examination of the Outdoor Casebooks, which describe the outcomes for women attended by St Helens midwives at home, will enable a comparison of home and hospital births attended by the same midwives with the same socio-economic group of women. This might shed some further light on the influence of the place of birth.

The issue not considered adequately by many authors is that it might be neither the type of birth attendant, nor the place of birth, but characteristics of the mother that contribute to outcomes – or indeed a complex interaction of all three factors. Developing hypotheses concerning one or other perspective may be too simplistic.

On other indices of the quality of maternity care, the midwife attendant appears to have made a large difference, with St Helens rates of forceps delivery, infections and infant mortality among the lowest in the country. Future research will explore the causes of maternal mortality among St Helens women, as they are well described in the case notes and provide an important reminder of the changes made in the identification and treatment of life-threatening conditions associated with childbearing.

TEARS AND SUTURES: INSCRIBING THE PERINEUM

One of the maternal outcomes recorded in the St Helens records was the state of the perineum. It was described as 'intact' or 'ruptured', with the extent of rupture described as 'first', 'second' or 'third degree'. Other descriptors used were 'laceration' or 'tear'. Records also noted whether there had been a repair of the rupture using 'sutures' or 'stitches', the number of stitches and sometimes the suture material (such as horsehair).

Our attention was caught by the fact that the descriptor 'episiotomy' was not used in any of the records. An episiotomy is an incision of the perineum during delivery to enlarge the vaginal orifice. According to Ian Graham's detailed study of episiotomy, its first recorded use was in the mid-eighteenth century. It was considered to be a procedure of last resort to save the perineum from rupturing when the usual non-surgical techniques (manual support of the perineum) had failed, or as an emergency procedure to save the life of the baby in cases where a rigid and unyielding perineum prevented its passage. The first description of the procedure Graham identified was in Sir Fielding Ould's midwifery text in 1742, where the recommendation was for two incisions, one either side of the fourchette. Later, its practice was endorsed by man-midwives Crede and Colpe in their 1884 analysis of 1,000 cases from their clinic in Leipzig, Germany, to (somewhat illogically) support their contention that episiotomy prevented perineal lacerations.[24]

The only Wellington St Helens description of such a procedure, although not named as episiotomy, occurs in the 1916 record. A healthy woman experienced what was considered an 'abnormal' labour 'due to a rigid perinaeum, necessitating two lateral incisions'. She went home with her baby on the fourteenth day 'in a satisfactory condition'. At this time obstetric authorities were still debating the appropriate use of episiotomy, with protagonists on both sides producing arguments either supporting its use to prevent the problematic spontaneous rupture that involved the anal sphincter, or against its use as it increased the risk of infection and 'childbed fever' as well as lengthy periods in hospital. With no agreement, it is not surprising that episiotomy was not liberally used in St Helens Wellington between 1907 and 1922.

When the complete record is entered on the database it will be possible to track when the procedure starts to be named as episiotomy and how its incidence increases or decreases over the ensuing decades as obstetrical 'fashion' dictated. This should provide useful information when critiquing the enduring belief in a rational-scientific sequential model of technological development in maternity care.

Similarly, an examination of suturing rates for women who had any tear or rupture of the perineum also suggests that decisions about this practice relied not necessarily on an agreed rationale but on some other factor, perhaps the professional preferences of the person attending the birth. The finding most suggestive of this is the marked spike in the suturing figures for 1914. There was a general increase in the percentage of women at St Helens Hospital recorded as having ruptures of the perineum over this period, from 17 per cent in 1908 to 26.13 per cent in 1920. The proportion of these women whose tears were sutured remained in the range of 5–12.5 per cent, except for an increase to 33.33 per cent in 1910 and 29.5 per cent in 1913. In 1914, however, the proportion rose to 65 per cent. A relatively low percentage of all women giving birth at St Helens that year were recorded as having ruptures or tears (18.09 per cent compared with 23.64 and 21.35 per cent in the two previous years, and 23.88 per cent the following year), yet nearly two-thirds of this 1914 group received sutures. What was unusual about that year that might explain it?

It was the midwife in attendance at the time of birth who made the decision about suturing. No difference was found in the suturing rates between the matron, Miss Inglis, or sub-matrons Sisters Maclean and Nutsey, who attended most of the births that year. The Department of Health's annual report covering 1914 suggested a possible explanation. Dr Agnes Bennett, the medical superintendent of St Helens Wellington, had left 'for service at the scene of war' at the beginning of April and the sub-matron, Veda Maclean, had left for war service in Samoa in August. A Dr Elliott was appointed as superintendent while Bennett was absent.[25] It seemed possible, therefore, that a change in personnel might account for the change in practice. A doctor was called in only for complicated births so their influence might have been more through policy than actual presence. The change in medical superintendent might have led to a change in policy regarding suturing. However, it is difficult to discern what this policy might have been. For example, a policy might have related to the severity of perineal tearing but further analysis did not support this. For those births in 1914 where the degree of rupture is recorded, no suturing trend can be discerned. First-degree tears were sutured (usually with one stitch) or left unsutured in equal numbers, the single second-degree tear recorded was left unsutured and two 'severe' ruptures were repaired with six stitches. An explanation for the 1914 incidence is therefore still to be discovered.

The Department of Health was also interested in this aspect of childbirth. In 1910 it began reporting a greater range of statistics from the combined St Helens Hospitals. Previously only live births, stillbirths, and maternal and infant mortality rates were reported. Between 1910 and 1914, the reports included statistics on 'operations' (such as induction, version, forceps and manual removal of the placenta), 'complications' (such as albuminuria, placenta praevia and eclampsia) and 'lacerated perinaeum'. Figures of perineal lacerations were recorded for primiparous and multiparous women and instrumental deliveries, as well as by the degree of laceration. The perineum was therefore inscribed with a bureaucratic as well as midwifery hand.[26]

Several other questions remain to be answered, for example, 'who was doing the suturing, with what, and were there any other treatments or complications?', and 'how does the rate of perineal tearing compare with today and what are the factors that might contribute to any difference?'

THE DESCRIPTIVE GAZE: BREASTS AND BREASTFEEDING

One of the first pieces of information to be recorded about each woman, in the 'Notes on the Case', was a description of her breasts. This was perhaps written on admission, when a comment on her general health was recorded. Most women (91.59 per cent) received a favourable comment and overwhelmingly the phrases used were 'mammae well developed' or 'breasts and nipples well developed'. Other terms included 'fairly' or 'moderately well developed', 'good' or 'excellent condition', 'quite normal' and 'well formed'. Descriptions that could be considered less favourable included 'small', 'not well developed', 'badly developed' or 'poorly developed', 'flat' and 'undersized'. Sometimes one breast received particular attention, as in 'one breast useless' or 'left breast well developed, right not'. Nipples were at times given a separate description, as in 'healthy', 'good condition', 'small', 'not well developed', 'inverted', 'flat' or 'retracted'. If the condition of the breast changed during the puerperium, for example if they became tender or cracked, this too was noted along with the treatment given.

This attention to and careful description of the development and condition of the breasts and nipples intrigued us. To Wood, as an historian, it was of interest as an indication of how midwives in the past understood their practice and what it encompassed. For Foureur, as a clinical professor in midwifery, it provided a contrast with current midwifery practice. Some midwives pay similar attention in antenatal visits to the condition of the breasts and nipples, whereas others make no such observations. By combining our perspectives we could see the potential this historical research could have in helping midwives today critique their own practice. Comparing the variations in practice now with the uniformity of scrutiny and recording in this hospital in the past offers midwives a basis for considering how they shape their understanding of their role and what they use as a basis for knowledge. If it was considered such an important aspect of practice in the past, why is it not today? Was there a rationale for doing it then? Has the basis of knowledge changed? Has the way we construct knowledge shifted?

Wood was also interested in what these descriptions might say about midwives' understanding of the 'good breast' and how this construction fits within a current cultural history of the breast. Marilyn Yalom's work, for example, traces the sacred, erotic, domestic, political, psychological, commercialized and medical constructions of the breast in history.[27] Exploring how midwives were constructing the notion of the 'good breast' in one New Zealand hospital in the early decades of the twentieth century adds a specific, localized example to this cultural history discussion. It should not be assumed, of course, that these descriptions recorded an accurate observation of each woman's breasts. The persistent use of the most common phrases might indicate a degree of habitual or routinized recording or, in perhaps a less critical light, the comfortable use of a convention of language that midwives brought with them to St Helens, or which they generated as a group while there, or which they were directed to use. We cannot tell who entered these descriptions in the records, whether it was the registered midwife in attendance or a midwife in training. Neither can we tell whether they created these descriptions themselves or were directed to use these conventions by the medical superintendent. Nevertheless, even a routinized recording, using a descriptive convention, offers a glimpse into the culture existing at St Helens Hospital in these years in which importance was placed on recording a descriptive statement about the woman's breasts.

While 'well developed' does not say a great deal about size or shape, both the description and its recording as the woman came in to give birth suggest that the good breast was one that had been well developed for a purpose – successful breastfeeding. As Yalom has noted, as a defining part of the female body the breast has been coded with both 'good' and 'bad' connotations through time, with the 'good' linked to its power to nourish infants or, allegorically, a political community. At St Helens Hospital, the 'good breast' was seemingly one large enough to contain adequate milk-producing tissue, so that it would produce a sufficient milk supply and deliver this to the infant through a well-protruding nipple. The breast was therefore inscribed with a solely nurturant function, an instrument for achieving the hospital's goal of sending healthy, suckling infants to their working-class Wellington homes. Breasts that did not inspire midwives' confidence became a site of intervention, with nipples rolled and massaged, cracks and fissures painted with sticky brown Benzoin and pumps applied to coax a reluctant milk supply. Establishing breastfeeding was the combined responsibility of the mother (to provide the well-functioning breast), the infant (to suckle effectively) and the midwife (to oversee and intervene efficiently).

This local interest in the breasts and breastfeeding was part of a wider, national and international interest. Rima Apple has provided a social history of infant feeding, 1890–1950 which focuses particularly on the US experience.[28] The changing ideas, issues and fashions there are reflected to a considerable extent in New Zealand. In the first decades of the twentieth century, the Department of Health's increasing concern for infant welfare, including nutrition, was evident in its annual reports. Between 1910 and 1914, along with the lacerated perineum statistics, the Department of Health reports included figures on 'inability to nurse', whether 'complete' or 'partial'.[29]

The reports suggested that only 1–2 per cent of women giving birth in all the St Helens Hospitals were completely unable to breastfeed, and 6–10 per cent were partially unable to do so. Reasons for this were carefully ascribed. Poor general health (such as anaemia, malnutrition or general debility), accompanying diseases and conditions (such as phthisis, chronic nephritis or influenza), conditions relating to childbirth (such as eclampsia, albuminuria or prematurity), the condition of the breast itself (such as 'defective breasts', inverted or retracted nipples, fissured nipples or mastitis), and low milk production were all listed as reasons. The 1912 report commented that a large number of women had been partially unable to nurse due to anaemia. Supplementary feeds were given twice a day to their babies and, in a congratulatory tone, the report noted that many were able to breastfeed completely by the third week. The Wellington records show that the mother might also be given a 'supplementary feed', as those unable to breastfeed successfully were given a proprietary preparation to increase the milk supply.

The St Helens Hospitals throughout the country therefore provided the government with the means to gather information about infant feeding and, at the local level, the midwives were the ones recording it. Whereas helping to establish successful breastfeeding would be seen as part of any midwife's scope of practice, the Wellington St Helens Hospital context provided an additional reason for their diligence in recording information about the breasts. Dr Agnes Bennett, the medical superintendent from 1908 until 1936, was keenly interested in the topic of breastfeeding and wrote a thesis on it for her MD from Edinburgh University in 1911.[30] Bennett's association with St Helens Hospital gave her ample opportunity to study breastfeeding in greater detail, with a ready-to-hand sample of mothers. No doubt the midwives' observations and recordings provided valuable material for her research.

Her authority to speak on this topic, however, had already been recognized. The Chief Medical Officer of the Department of Health, Dr James Mason, who was keenly interested in infant feeding, asked her to write a new pamphlet on the subject to help mothers understand its significance and to provide practical advice.[31] This pamphlet, *Baby's Welfare*, was published in 1907. It stressed the importance of breastfeeding, gave practical tips for managing problems such as flat nipples, a slow milk supply or the baby's reluctance to suckle, instructed mothers on how artificial feeding should be managed if absolutely necessary, and covered other helpful topics such as weight gain, weaning and minor ailments that might afflict either mother or infant.[32] The pamphlet was published in the same year, however, that Dr Frederic Truby King established the Society for Promoting the Health of Women and Children. Concerned particularly with encouraging effective infant feeding, it quickly became an influential New Zealand institution generally known as the Plunket Society.[33] As the strong influential force behind it, Truby King considered himself the authority, and therefore the rightful national spokesman, on infant feeding. His urging of mothers to feed their infants at regular intervals had as much to do with instilling discipline as ensuring effective nutrition.[34] If mothers were not able to breastfeed, he advocated the use of his carefully devised process for producing 'humanized milk'. Bennett's pamphlet contained similar information but was clearly seen by Truby King as a challenge to his authority and position in the field. He criticized its contents and, immediately after being made Director of the Division of Child Welfare within the Department of Health in 1920, he pulled it from circulation.[35]

St Helens Hospital therefore had a significant role in the development of knowledge about infant feeding, through the midwives' careful observations and recordings. With Bennett's official position as medical superintendent, it also provided a clinical base for research, as well as an institutional context for arguing her authority in the field. Truby King's challenge to this, however, meant that St Helens Hospital became a locus not only for constructing knowledge but also for contesting it.

A closer analysis of the patient records could consider many other questions. In relation to infant feeding, for example, the proportion of babies given supplementary feeds and the changing nature of supplementary feeds over time could be calculated; in turn, the impact of commercial production of infant feeding mixtures could be investigated and the whole set in an international context. The maternal position in infant feeding could be further investigated by exploring the relationships between the mother's general health status, age and parity, and ability to breastfeed; similarly the impact on ability to breastfeed of receiving drugs during labour and birth could be pursued. Any of these features might be associated with the socio-economic status of the location of their Wellington homes.

CONCLUSION

The Wellington St Helens archive offers a unique record of one institution that delivered maternity care for working-class women in New Zealand. Analysis of its birth-related records, 1907–22, provides distinct advantages for both historical and epidemiological lines of enquiry. For the historian, the archive allows a local study that can comment on contemporary national trends, providing examples of these or describing exceptions. For both the historian and the epidemiologist, it provides evidence to support or challenge past and current ideas about trends and causes of adverse health outcomes for childbearing women. For example, reasons for differences in maternal mortality rates according to the type of attendant, place of birth and socio-economic class, proposed by contemporary commentators or current historians, can be reviewed in light of the results from one specific institution. The evidence from the Wellington St Helens Hospital, although related to a relatively small number of women, is even more important because the hospital offered a degree of control over frequently occurring confounding variables, as in these years it provided a service delivered predominantly by midwives and only to working-class women. In this way it acted as an historical 'living laboratory'.

Similarly, it offers current healthcare providers, particularly midwives, useful insights into models of care delivery that contributed to safe maternity services in the past. Changing techniques of care, for example in relation to suturing, can also be discerned. Further analysis of the archive and related primary sources, such as government reports and contemporary scientific literature, could determine the extent to which these changes in practice were based on scientific evidence, obstetrical 'fashion' or individual professional preference.

Its case notes allow glimpses into the realities of women's childbirth experiences and changing midwifery practices. For the cultural historian, these case notes are also a rich source for discerning how one group of midwives created and shared ideas about practice. The aspects of childbirth, specific complications and treatments, captured in the records, offer a glimpse into the ways the process of childbirth and the post-partum period were constructed in a system of shared meanings. Although precisely who recorded the notes and who determined the language conventions for them is unclear, the notes reveal the way the childbearing woman's body was inscribed with meaning. For example, ideas about the 'good breast', effective nipple and productive mother, and changing constructions of the lacerated perineum as problematic or benign, emerge from an analysis of the case notes. Similarly, the Department of Health's requirement for increasingly detailed reports on perineal lacerations show how the perineum was inscribed by both bureaucrat and midwife.

The St Helens Hospitals were effective in providing safe maternity care for working-class women in New Zealand. The Department of Health held them as the exemplar of best practice, with significantly better outcomes for women on indices such as forceps, puerperal sepsis and infant mortality rates than other places of childbirth, whether hospital or home. Only on rates of maternal mortality is Wellington St Helens Hospital nearly equivalent to the national rate, although this requires a more finely grained analysis. Analysis of its birth-related records enables a midwife–epidemiologist to assess the relevance of this historical example to the present-day community of birthing women, with the aim of improving maternity care outcomes. For the historian, it offers a significant single source, an almost complete record of childbirth at one important institution delivering a state maternity service to working-class women in New Zealand.

ACKNOWLEDGEMENTS

We are grateful to Abbey McDonald for her conscientious, skilful and good-humoured assistance in this research. We are also grateful to Victoria University of Wellington for two Faculty of Humanities and Social Sciences grants, and to Capital and Coast Health for their grant, to support both phases of the database development.

NOTES

1 During the 1920s particularly, St Helens Hospitals had the lowest rates for puerperal sepsis, forceps deliveries and, from 1927, maternal mortality of all hospitals in New Zealand providing a maternity service. See, for example, P. Mein Smith, *Maternity in Dispute, New Zealand 1920–1939,* Wellington: Historical Publications Branch, Department of Internal Affairs, 1986, pp. 61–2, 72, 77–8, 118.

2 Mein Smith, *Maternity in Dispute*; J. Donley, *Save the Midwife*, Auckland: New Women's Press, 1986; E. Papps and M. Olssen, *Doctoring Childbirth and Regulating Midwifery in New Zealand: A Foucauldian Perspective*, Palmerston North: Dunmore Press, 1997; C. Parkes, 'The impact of medicalization of New Zealand's maternity services on women's experience of childbirth, 1904–1937', in L. Bryder (ed.),

A Healthy Country: Essays on the Social History of Medicine in New Zealand, Wellington: Bridget Williams Books, 1991, pp. 165–80.

3   J. O. C. Neill, *Grace Neill, the Story of a Noble Woman,* Christchurch: N. M. Peryer, 1961. Although this account is written by Grace Neill's son, her role in the development of this legislation is not overestimated. J. O. C. Neill states that Grace Neill's suggestion for the name St Helens was made during a personal interview with Seddon and that it was an inspired idea to ensure his support for the legislation. A 1905 letter from Neill to Seddon, however, says simply that 'a name had to be found for them, and St Helens seemed appropriate'. Letter from Neill to Seddon, 2 February 1905, Inspector-General's Office, Wellington, held at Archives New Zealand.

4   The first baby born there, on 17 June 1905, was named Richard John, in honour of the Premier.

5   *Appendices to the Journals of the House of Representatives,* 1906, H-22, p. 3.

6   See, for example, *Appendices to the Journals,* 1907, H-22 p. 3; 1908, H-22 p. 9; 1909, H-22 p. 11; 1910, H-22 p. 11; 1911, H-31, p. 80; 1912, H-31 p. 22; 1913, H-31, p. 14.

7   H. Jellett, *A Short Practice of Midwifery for Nurses,* London: J. and A. Churchill, 1929. T. F. Corkhill, *Lectures on Midwifery and Infant Care: A New Zealand Course,* Wellington: Coulls Somerville Wilkie, 1932.

8   These reforms are described in Mein Smith, *Maternity in Dispute.*

9   See, for example, *Appendices to the Journals,* 1926, H-31, p. 23 and p. 25. See also Mein Smith, *Maternity in Dispute,* pp. 64–6.

10 By 1935, however, 78 per cent were in maternity hospitals, with 8 per cent at St Helens Hospitals. Mein Smith, *Maternity in Dispute,* p. 1.

11 Ministry of Health, *Report on Maternity 1999,* Wellington: Ministry of Health, 2001.

12 K. James, P. J. Steer, C. P. Weiner and B. Gonik, *High Risk Pregnancy Management Options,* 2nd edn, London: W. B. Saunders, 1999.

13 The European infant mortality rates (deaths of infants under one year per 1,000 live births) were 68.46 for 1907–11; 52.50 for 1912–16; 48.04 for 1917–21; and 41.17 for 1922–26. F. S. Maclean, *Challenge for Health: A History of Public Health in New Zealand,* Wellington: R. E. Owen, Government Printer, 1964, p. 176.

14 Mein Smith, *Maternity in Dispute,* p. 5.

15 I. Loudon, 'Midwives and the quality of maternal care', in H. Marland and A. M. Rafferty (eds), *Midwives, Society and Childbirth,* London: Routledge, 1997, pp. 180–200.

16 Ibid., pp. 183, 184.

17 Ibid., Table 8.4, Maternal mortality rates in various countries around 1920, and the usual attendants at normal births, p. 192.

18 *Appendices to the Journals,* 1928, H-31, p. 9. The entry notes that 1920 was a peak year with an undue proportion of first births, the result of returned soldier marriages, and that statisticians regarded first births as more at risk of fatality than subsequent births.

19 Loudon, 'Midwives and quality', p. 191.

20 Ibid., p. 185.

21 We have aggregated the data for this time period to account for yearly fluctuations in maternal deaths, as some official government records did in that time.

22 Mein Smith, *Maternity in Dispute,* pp. 19–20.

23 See, for example, *Appendices to the Journals,* 1909, H-22, p. 16; 1910, H-22 p. 11; 1911, H-31, p. 83; 1914, H-31 p. 12; 1915, H-31, p. 7; 1923, H-31 p. 32.

24 I. D. Graham, *Episiotomy: Challenging Obstetric Interventions,* Oxford: Blackwell Science, 1997. For further discussion of the history of episiotomy, see, for example, S. B. Thacker and D. H. Banta, 'Benefits and risks of episiotomy: An interpretative review of the English language literature, 1860–1980', *Obstetrical and Gynecological Survey,* 1983, Vol. 38, (6), pp. 322–338; C. East and J. Webster, 'Episiotomy at the

Royal Women's Hospital, Brisbane: A comparison of practices in 1986 and 1992', *Midwifery,* 1995, Vol. 11, pp. 195–200.

25   *Appendices to the Journals,* 1915, H-31, p. 7.

26   Ibid., 1910, H-22 p. 15; 1911, H-31 p. 82; 1912, H-31 p. 24; 1913, H-31 p. 16; 1914, H-31 p. 11. From 1915 these statistics are not reported, probably because the length of all government reports was severely curtailed during World War I and did not really expand again until the 1930s.

27   M. Yalom, *A History of the Breast,* New York: Alfred A. Knopf, 1997.

28   R. D. Apple, *Mothers and Medicine: A Social History of Infant Feeding, 1890–1950,* Madison: University of Wisconsin Press, 1987.

29   *Appendices to the Journals,* 1910, H-22 pp. 15–16; 1911, H-31 pp. 81–3; 1912, H-31 pp. 24–5; 1913, H-31 pp. 16–18; 1914, H-31 pp. 11–12.

30   C. and C. Manson, *Doctor Agnes Bennett,* London: Michael Joseph, 1960, pp. 67–8.

31   Derek Dow, *Safeguarding the Public Health: A History of the New Zealand Department of Health,* Wellington: Victoria University Press, 1995, p. 65.

32   Agnes Bennett, *Baby's Welfare: Practical Hints to Mothers,* Wellington: Public Health Department, 1907, held at Alexander Turnbull Library, Wellington.

33   Lady Plunket was patron of the society. For a short account of its history, see Lynne Giddings, 'Royal New Zealand Plunket Society', in Anne Else (ed.), *Women Together: a History of Women's Organisations in New Zealand,* Wellington: Historical Branch, Department of Internal Affairs and Daphne Brasell Associates Press, 1993, pp. 257–61. For a more detailed history, see Linda Bryder, *A Voice for Mothers: the Plunket Society and Infant Welfare 1907–2000,* Auckland: Auckland University Press, 2003.

34   For further on this point, see Erik Olssen, 'Truby King and the Plunket Society: An analysis of a prescriptive ideology', *New Zealand Journal of History,* 1981, Vol. 15, (1), pp. 3–23.

35   Philippa Mein Smith says that the pamphlet Truby King removed from circulation was one entitled *Domestic Hygiene.* However, as this pamphlet was published in 1921 and Truby King was appointed in 1920, it is likely to be this earlier pamphlet, *Baby's Welfare,* that was withdrawn. It contained the 'dietary information similar to that found in Plunket literature' to which Mein Smith refers, whereas the later one does not. As Mein Smith points out, the two doctors had previously argued publicly about higher education for women. Mein Smith, *Maternity in Dispute,* p. 19.

12 Common working ground

Joan E. Lynaugh

Modern nursing emerged as a distinct entity only during the last 150 years or so in Germany, England, Scandinavia and North America. It became an idea so formidable, and so seemingly inevitable, that nursing now encircles the world. The nursing I speak of is the modern, recognizable, standardized occupation of nursing. In turn, modern nursing rests, however uneasily, on a time-immemorial idea of nursing or mutual aid among humans that seems to date from ancient, even prehistoric, times. Whether modern or ancient, nursing deals with birth and death, health and illness; it is ubiquitous and essential. Those who study the history of nursing have a broad field indeed, and several audiences for their musings.

America's early nurse historian, Lavinia L. Dock, focused in on one of those audiences in 1907. As a determined professionalizer, she saw history as a means and a tool to make nurses self-conscious of their own identity and potential power. She spoke directly to them. 'Only in the light of history can she (the modern nurse) clearly see how closely her own calling is linked with the general conditions of education and of liberty that obtain – as they rise, she rises, and as they sink, she falls'.[1] As historian Sioban Nelson explains so well, Dock and other promulgators of her traditional view and use of history were, indeed, very effective in creating a collective self-image and group identification for the new field.[2]

But, encouraged by Nelson's argument, I am more interested in discussing one of the other audiences historians of nursing must consider. That audience is ourselves. An international history of nursing cannot be realized unless there is an international body of scholars. To return once more to an early historian of nursing, let me quote American Adelaide Nutting writing in the International Council of Nurses *Bulletin* in 1924; 'we must . . . find somewhere, between the extremes of thought and opinion, the best common working ground'.[3] In this brief essay I consider three elements that I believe are fundamental as we historians think about our own 'common working ground.'

First, it seems to me that certain historical subjects are of universal importance – making them attractive to study and likely to build the field. For now I will suggest eight subject areas from my own experience. No doubt there are many other possibilities that will intrigue scholars.

Next, to build a body of scholarship, we need to be both cognizant of and sensitive to distracting issues and pitfalls, as individual historians from different cultures and world views work together. It goes without saying that the work we do must be intellectually responsible in history and meet those quality standards. But, it is also true that those of us who are nurses must expect and be prepared to defend our subject and our findings within our own profession.

Finally, I will propose what I think are some important and long-lasting advantages for the discipline of nursing history if we find that an international, communicating body of scholars in nursing history can be achieved.

EIGHT SUBJECTS FOR STUDY

Nursing and the state

The wide variation and complexity found in the many ways nursing relates to the state form a context of pressing interest to historians. We recognize that nursing–state relationships range from regulatory and legislative negotiations and rules, to political alliances, to patriotic responses when state sovereignty is threatened, to occupational self-identity, and might include ideological preferences and positions. In our 1999 study of the International Council of Nurses (ICN), for example, we found the ways nurses conceived of their linkages to the state endlessly fascinating and constantly changing.[4] The design and constitution of the ICN was, of course, itself a reflection of the emerging nation–state political forms of the nineteenth and twentieth centuries. In 1900, the ICN founders were certain that the best means of ensuring a firm basis for their new profession must be the establishment of single national nurse organizations, each recognized as the standard setter by its respective country. Then, the ICN sought to bring these national nurse organizations together in a federation hoping, thereby, to forge a strong international nursing organization. Implicit in this design were two ideas, or perhaps two unexamined assumptions. First, nursing should play an integral role in the infrastructure of the modern state. The second assumption was that the best route to professional recognition was via state-sanctioned legal status. These decisions by the founders of organized nursing meant that an essentially private matter, the relationship between nurse and patient, would, from then on, be embedded in the larger context of organized nursing and the state.

Another way this public role becomes especially evident is when it comes to nursing and war. The dramatic images of the Crimea and the two world wars, the romance of women nurses helping soldiers whatever their uniform, and the societal reward accruing to nursing when it is able to play a patriotic role, all work to draw attention to military matters and nursing. In some sense, as former ICN President Annie Goodrich dramatically proclaimed before the ICN in 1925, 'nursing germinated in the heart of destruction'.[5] Perhaps as our historical scholarship in nursing develops in this genre, we will focus less on romance and more on analytic work. An excellent example is Anne Summers' in-depth exploration of British nurses in the late nineteenth and early twentieth centuries.[6] A more recent and darker example of the interplay between nurses and the state is starkly portrayed in Bronwyn Rebekah McFarland-Icke's *Nurses in Nazi Germany: Moral Choice in History*.[7]

There is a growing body of scholarship exploring this overall subject of nursing and the state. In this book, for example, authors Hvalvik and Hackmann treat the matter from different perspectives; each importantly adds to our growing comprehension of the positive and negative interdependence of nursing and country. In fact, a great many histories of nursing use a particular country as a frame. My own work with Barbara Brush is an example of this tendency.[8] But there is a lot of historical room for broader views, especially those that step back from the focus on a single country and contemplate regional or global implications and outcomes of various nurse–state arrangements.

Religious influences

Similarly, turning to another subject, we can easily see how rich historical studies of religion and nursing can be. There are some very encouraging recent examples, including the work of Sioban Nelson, Asa Andersson and Katrin Schultheiss.[9] Andersson's close examination of the influence of Lutheran beliefs on the evolution of organized nursing in Sweden might be a template for other studies. New research on the work of religious orders who nursed, such as that of Barbra Mann Wall, illuminates the culture–religion intersection as religious women worked in various parts of the world.[10] There are, however, remarkably few fully realized studies of nurse missionaries, considering the popularity of that calling among nurses during the nineteenth and twentieth centuries. The old cliché, 'born in the church, bred in the military' does have some valid connections to the history of nursing in some parts of the world, but not all. What will historians of nursing in Thailand, India, Jordan and Russia tell us about religious beliefs and nursing?

Economics and nursing

Modern nursing developed in the context of the worldwide spread of industrialization and an increasingly cash-based economy. Inherently, the occupation of modern nursing involves transferring part of the family, tribe or village care-taking responsibility to a paid worker, a stranger, whose work is somehow deemed and guaranteed to be trustworthy. Whether this transaction took place universally, and whether, as I have implied, it was a consequence of industrialization is worth investigating. How paid nursing was constructed and conducted in different parts of the world is poorly understood. Even in countries where active scholarship in the history of nursing is quite developed, the economic history of the field remains underexplored. Perhaps that is so because we are more intrigued by issues of gender and power. Or, perhaps we, as historians, don't reflect much on nursing as 'paid work'. For instance, there is not a large body of work exploring the tense and tenuous relationship between trade unions and nursing. Considering the vital importance of the nursing workforce to the operations of modern health systems, historians certainly can contribute to a clearer understanding of the issues. We know that nursing is very important in modern economies. But there is much to understand and interpret about how and why nursing functioned in the economies of the last two centuries.

Social welfare

Closely tying together the economic history of nursing, the relationship of nursing to the state, and the history of religion and nursing is the matter of social welfare and modern nursing. How is the welfare of the larger society articulated and determined in different times, places, political systems and economies? Has nursing been part of this determination? If so, was nursing's concept of social welfare linked to health? Have individual nurses' roles been coercive, protective or supportive of the recipient of social welfare? Again, the partial transfer of the traditional social responsibilities of the family and/or relational group to outside private or public entities influenced the history of nursing in some countries. How universal and influential was this connection between nursing and social welfare? What meaning does it have for international nursing or for the idea of nursing at all? Historian Anne Marie Rafferty's critical reappraisal of the history of nursing in the UK is a good example of a sophisticated approach to thinking about this complex, interlinking historical context so influential on today's nursing in some parts of the world.[11]

Gender

Once the influence of the women's movement of the 1970s began to permeate academia and generate scholarship on women and history, it was only a matter of time until the history of nursing would begin to be examined through the lens of gender. The impact of the development of women's studies on the history of nursing is very visible in certain countries. In the USA the most influential history of nursing is certainly Susan Reverby's *Ordered to Care: The Dilemma of American Nursing, 1850–1945*.[12] Historian Reverby made the argument that nurses were obligated to care in a society that refused to value caring and that training for nursing was based on ideas of women's duties, not women's rights. Her book resonated with her 1987 audience. During the next decade a small but influential new history of nursing began to develop, offering insights into the history of women and relationships between men and women.[13] Explorations of the impact of nineteenth-century nursing reforms on men in nursing and the part played by men in modern nursing warrant further study.[14] Studying the history of nursing using the lens of gender will go a long way towards revealing and interpreting the tapestry of cultural preferences and variations in the universe of nursing.

To round out my admittedly personal list of the nursing history subjects I think have universal applicability, I will add three connected subjects; these are modern scientific thinking, changing medical ideas and nursing knowledge.

Scientific thinking

Surely the most dramatic intellectual change in the last 300 years is the wide-spread adoption of scientific thinking and experimentation as the preferred basis for authoritative decision making. Beginning around 1700 or so, people gradually began to turn to scientific thinking instead of relying on revealed truth or tradition when dealing with certain problems, for instance, improving agriculture, navigation, medicine and manufacturing. Armed with new and different sources of renewable knowledge, people began to reject the authority of religious or God-ordained leaders. At the same time, they reduced their dependence on tradition and tradition bearers.

Measuring its impact on governments, social contracts, economies, education and every other facet of life, the influence of scientific thinking was especially prevalent in the Western world. Science-based authority spread throughout the world during the twentieth century. That is not to say that Western ideas necessarily prevailed over older cultures but, instead, it is to say that the ways that humans interpret the world are everywhere influenced by scientific thinking. Thus, this process of problem identification, data gathering, hypothesis formation and hypothesis testing now permeates many, if not all, areas of modern life. Nowhere is this more evident than in care of the sick and our vision of health.

Medical changes

Modern nursing history shows the links between the rise of scientific thinking, the subsequent changes in medical ideas and the impact of these forces on the formation and development of nursing. Medicine underwent extensive change during the eighteenth and nineteenth centuries as long-held medical theories fell victim to testing. As was true of science in general, changes in actual medical practice were gradual and care continued to be influenced by other forces such as class relationships, social responsibility and personal style. But, ultimately, ideas about disease changed, and with that change came progressive and sweeping changes in therapeutics. As historian Charles Rosenberg notes, the new medical point of view 'implied the possibility of turning each ailment and each organ into a subject of ordered and systematic investigation'.[15] Promulgated first in Germany and Scotland, and then in France, new medical ideas and knowledge transformed the practice of medicine between 1800 and 1900.

For this new practice of medicine to flourish, and indeed it did come to flourish over the nineteenth and into the twentieth century, hospitals became increasingly important. Scientific medicine and, more important, the emerging practice of surgery needed the accoutrements of the hospital. It became more and more difficult to practise medicine or nursing entirely in the patient's home. The advent and application of anaesthesia and antiseptic techniques called for centralization of facilities and knowledge about how to use them. As historians of modern nursing know, gathering patients together in hospitals proved problematic. Reliable and informed caretakers were essential to prevent chaos and relieve suffering. The modern nurse appeared on the scene with the modern hospital.

It was not just changes in medical thought and practice, however, that inspired the spread of the hospital. Changes in the economies of Europe and America, northern Africa, Japan, Australia and parts of South America led to population shifts and urbanization. Dislocated populations turned to institutions for relief during illness and the hospital became more than just a hospice for travellers or a shelter for the indigent. It began to be a vital and quite ubiquitous social institution. The development and spread of modern, secular nursing, often modelled after the nursing of earlier religious nursing orders and also based on domestic ideals of the nineteenth century, made the hospital possible. The institutionalization of care of the sick, as described here, was not a universal phenomenon. It was tightly linked to urbanization, as noted above, but it was also fundamentally dependent on sufficient social affluence to make it possible for the populace to invest in care of the dependent and ill.

Nursing knowledge

New knowledge from biology, chemistry and pathology markedly affected the development of modern nursing. The advent of the germ theory and its eventual acceptance, new ideas about diet and cleanliness as ways to fend off illness, and a growing belief in general education of the public, all served to support public health. In some parts of the world, especially where urbanization and immigration were widespread, nurses began to be employed as agents to spread these new ideas of collective health.[16]

Nursing knowledge can be an elusive subject because, as it has developed, its tendency is to be inclusive, rather than to reduce questions to the small segments normative in scientific thinking. Nurses learn, among other things, an array of domestic and personal care skills, human interaction skills, science, including the social sciences, application and interpretation of technology, various medical skills and theories, data collection, management and interpretation, applications of probability, and system administration. Nursing knowledge is applied during reciprocal interactions with individual people and groups. Novice nurses learn nursing in direct and intimate ways, by caring for people. Nurses learn from written sources and other media, by experimenting and by imitating experts. As is true of most professionals who provide direct personal services, nurses also learn from their patients.

Historians are interested in various facets of nursing knowledge, including the vast changes in its scope and depth over time. One subject of interest is the awkward 'fit' of nursing knowledge in the major knowledge schemes of the twentieth century, especially those dominated by controlled scientific studies. The fit is awkward because nurses find it difficult to reduce some of their clinical questions to completely testable hypotheses. Think, for example, of caring for the dying, responding to emergencies, or supporting a patient's spiritual needs. On the other hand, nurses creatively generate new knowledge and re-frame clinical care issues to solve them in the context where they occur. Think of the matter of preventing the spread of infection among institutionalized people or educating women in pregnancy prevention. The intellectual development of nursing, and the subsequent rapid changes in education for nurses, offers a rich field for historical study and interpretation.

These subjects – nursing and the state, religious influences, the economy and nursing, social welfare, gender, and scientific thinking, medical changes and nursing knowledge – offer an ambitious and expandable agenda for scholarship. Readers should add other subjects – race and ethnicity and technology might well be on my own next list.

THINGS TO WORRY ABOUT

Now, I want to suggest a few cautions or things to worry about as we move forward. While contemplating this matter of finding 'common working ground', I can't help but reflect on how easy it is for each of us to mistake our own ways for universal ways. By making this list of subjects for study, for example, I run the risk of a kind of 'historical imperialism', an attempt to predetermine the scholarly agenda. Moreover, I am an American and, by necessity, can know the world only within that limitation. We are all the products of our own environment and experience. Indeed, it would be remarkable if we did not think the way *we* know must be the best way. Or, to take this point a bit further, we might, as historian Thomas Haskell warns, 'mistake our own ways for universal ways and experience the 'Other' as an imperfect approximation of ourselves, always obstinately falling short of the good, as currently and locally understood'.[17]

It is crucial to recall that the conclusions drawn from a case study, however well done or seemingly central, cannot be universal. Still, as we consider pursuing an international approach to the study of the history of nursing we can use our historians' skills to fortify ourselves against the dual risks of trivializing through superficiality and suppressing important differences.

It is our good fortune that we have the tools at hand. Historical interpretation and analysis means placing events, institutions and people in the broad context in which they happened or lived. We find and evaluate evidence, frame questions and apply tests of logic. We form historical concepts and use historical exposition and narrative to create and interpret the history of the event, institution, person or idea. Our fundamental task is to make reliable evidence (once found) yield maximum meaning within its own context and to explain the 'nature' of the events, institution, person or idea.

Our task is to try to explain unpredictable events in retrospect. History is, of course, non-experimental and so it allows study of the idiosyncratic. Most important, history deals with particular happenings; good history means including all the evidence and context around those happenings. Thus, history is like real life, it is contingent. Science necessarily tries to control contingencies, but we historians must include and acknowledge them in our analyses. Still, history, like science, must be of consequence, revealing what the world needs to know.[18] As can be gathered from what has been said so far, I, for one, firmly believe that the world needs to know what we can tell them.

WHAT CAN BE GAINED BY AN INTERNATIONAL APPROACH TO THE HISTORY OF NURSING?

As I think about the implications of creating a recognizable connection among scholars of the history of nursing around the world, that is, creating a universe of such scholars, a cluster of opportunities come to mind.

First, membership, recognition and reputation among a recognized group give the individual scholar linkages beyond his or her local situation. We all work in schools, agencies or organizations with certain missions and assigned tasks. But, to verify our work and to validate its authenticity, we need an audience of peers. In countries where nursing history associations exist these needs can, to some extent, be met. But the number of such associations is few and they are, of course, bounded by their national character. In any case, our field is so small that enhancing our connectedness carries obvious benefits in terms of mutual support.

Another benefit of an international collective of scholars is that it will create conditions for heightened creativity and critical thinking. We have all experienced the stimulation and new insights gained from hearing another viewpoint on a familiar topic. We know that entirely new research ideas can be generated when opportunities for exchange are broadened.

We all need the freedom to think and write. At the same time, as a community of the competent, we need to expose ourselves to criticism and review. We need to ensure for our various audiences that the scholarship we produce is authoritative.

The history of nursing attracts and interests many people. But those actually engaged in researching and writing history constitute a tiny fraction of all nurses and an almost equally small fraction of historians. It is fair to say that we experience a more or less constant case of 'strangeness' or perhaps even 'invisibility'. Finding ways to participate in a coalition of historians around the world would do much to relieve that nagging sense of not being seen or heard.

And, finally, in important ways, an international group of scholars lends a certain identity to all of its participants. Such a group offers a point of reference, a name, and a shared meaning for the individual scholar who works within it.

CONCLUSION

The chapters included in this publication validate our potential for taking the next steps to universally shared scholarship and, indeed, this book and the conference that inspired it are important examples of our future. Technology is on our side as well. Certainly the internet enables rapid, detailed and rich communications between historians. The emergence of the new history of nursing, which we saw in the later decades of the twentieth century, will surely mature, grow and help us better comprehend the connected, interdependent world of the twenty-first century.

NOTES

1   A. Nutting and L.L. Dock, *A History of Nursing,* Vol. 1, New York: G. P. Putnam's Sons, 1907, p. v.

2   S. Nelson, 'The fork in the road: nursing history versus the history of nursing', *Nursing History Review*, 2002, Vol. 10, pp. 175–88.

3   A. Nutting quoted in B. L. Brush and M. Stuart, 'Unity amidst difference: The ICN project and writing international nursing history', *Nursing History Review*, 1994, Vol. 2, pp. 191–203.

4   B. L. Brush and J. E. Lynaugh (eds), *Nurses of all Nations: A History of the International Council of Nurses, 1899–1999,* Philadelphia, PA: Lippincott, Williams and Wilkins, 1999. Contributing authors include N. Tomes, M. Stuart, A. M. Rafferty and G. Boschma.

5   A. W. Goodrich, *The Social and Ethical Significance of Nursing – A Series of Addresses* (reprint edition), New Haven, CT: Yale University School of Nursing, 1973, p. 204.

6   A. Summers, *Angels and Citizens: British Women as Military Nurses, 1854–1914,* London: Routledge, 1988.

7   B. R. McFarland-Icke, *Nurses in Nazi Germany – Moral Choice in History*, Princeton, NJ: Princeton University Press, 1999.

8   J. E. Lynaugh and B. L. Brush, *American Nursing: from Hospitals to Health Systems*, Cambridge, MA: Blackwell Publishers, 1996.

9   A. Andersson, 'To work in the garden of God: The Swedish Nursing Association and the concept of the calling, 1909–1933', *Nursing History Review*, 2002, Vol. 10, 3–19; S. Nelson, *Say Little, Do Much: Nursing, Nuns, and Hospitals in the Nineteenth Century,* Philadelphia: University of Pennsylvania Press, 2001 and, K. Schulththeiss, *Bodies and Souls: Politics and the Professionalization of Nursing in France, 1880–1922,* Cambridge, MA: Harvard University Press, 2001.

10 For instance, see Nelson *Say Little Do much,* and B. Mann-Wall, 'Courage to care: The Sisters of the Holy Cross in the Spanish-American War', *Nursing History Review*, 1995, Vol. 3, pp. 55–77.

11 A. M. Rafferty, *The Politics of Nursing Knowledge*, London: Routledge, 1996.

12 S. Reverby, *Ordered to Care: the Dilemma of American nursing, 1850–1945,* Cambridge: Cambridge University Press, 1987.

13 This is a growing and rich source of literature. A few examples help to indicate the range. P. O'Brien (D'Antonio), 'All a woman's life can bring': The domestic roots of nursing in Philadelphia, 1830–1885', *Nursing Research*, 1987, Vol. 36, pp. 12–17, L. E. Sabin, 'Unheralded nurses: male care givers in the nineteenth century South', *Nursing History Review*, 1997. Vol. 5, pp. 131–48, and M. Sandelowski, *Devices and Desires: Gender, Technology, and American Nursing,* Chapel Hill, NC: The University of North Carolina Press, 2000.

14 G. Boschma, 'The gender specific role of male nurses in Dutch asylums: 1890–1910', *International History of Nursing Journal*, 1999. Vol. 4, pp. 13–19.

15 C. E. Rosenberg, *The Care of Strangers: the Rise of America's Hospital System*, New York: Basic Books, Inc., 1987, p. 83.

16 K. Buhler-Wilkerson, *No Place like Home: a History of Nursing and Home Care in the United States,* Baltimore, MD: The Johns Hopkins University Press, 2001.

17 T. L. Haskell, *Objectivity is not Neutrality: Explanatory Schemes in History*, Baltimore, MD: The Johns Hopkins University Press, 1998, p. 281.

18 J. E. Lynaugh, 'Editorial', *Nursing History Review*, 1998, Vol. 6, n.p.

Index